Retrain Your Brain
CRPS

Complex Regional Pain Syndrome

Carol Charland

Revised Edition 2023

COPYRIGHT 2023 Carol Charland – All Rights Reserved

This is the creative property of Carol Charland. No part of this book may be reproduced in any manner without written permission by Carol Charland. No part of this creative work may be infringed upon by others for financial gain by photocopying, broadcasting or reproducing.

www.carolcharland.com

Dedication

To My Grandson Garrett,

Who gave me the strength to continue through some of my darkest pain-filled days. He brightens my days and fills my life with heartfelt joy. This is for you Garrett, to inspire you to be all you can be, there is nothing you cannot achieve in life, reach for the stars and grab your dreams.
Love Meme, xoxo

With My Gratitude

Dr. Pradeep Chopra, MD Pain management specialist and expert in the field of CRPS

I will forever be grateful to Dr Chopra for his expertise in diagnosing my CRPS. I went 9 years undiagnosed in horrific pain before I met Dr Chopra. It was his effective treatment protocols that gave me my life back from the grip of CRPS pain. Through my healing journey, I found a new life purpose of helping others with chronic pain. I would not be doing the work I am doing today as an advocate for CRPS Awareness and most importantly as a CAM Pain Management Practitioner helping people with chronic pain if not for Dr Chopra. I am forever grateful.

With My Gratitude

Mr. Jim Broatch and the RSDSA Organization

I would like to thank Mr. Jim Broatch and the RSDSA Organization who extended a helping hand during my darkest days of CRPS. They were instrumental in getting me the expert medical attention that facilitated my healing process.

The RSDSA organization is dedicated to CRPS Awareness and helping people with CRPS~RSD find the resources they need to live a better life. www.rsds.org

RSDSA is a non-profit organization on Amazon's charitable donation list. When purchasing my books, please consider RSDSA as your preferred charity.

5 Star Reviews By CRPS Patients

The Results After The 30-Day Program

"I have CRPS of the right hand after a wrist fracture on March 26 and surgery on April 2. I have completed the 30 day "Retrain the Brain" program. (I have included before and after pictures). The swelling is down and the discoloration has improved. I still have pain but it is reduced. There has been no change in mobility. I listen to the recording every night when I go to bed. The first 3 nights, it increased my anxiety level and I could not complete the sessions. However, on the 4th night, I fell asleep about half way through the recording. Now I fall asleep quickly and soundly.

Overall, at the end of the 30-day program, my hand has improved and I am able to get a good night's rest. I am going to continue listening to the daily recording"

-Rosie B

5 Star Reviews By CRPS Patients

A Wealth of Information

"Carol has written a multi-faceted book that every person with CRPS should have in his/her treatment tool kit.

This book paves the way for readers to incorporate well explained concepts into their lives; first by reading about the concept then completing exercises that reinforce the learning. The strength of the mind-body connection is woven throughout the book. From techniques focused on reducing pain and improving self-image to creating an inner sanctuary, capitalizing on the brain's plasticity and much more, there is something for everyone in this gem of a book"

- Deb B

5 Star Reviews By CRPS Patients

A Great Tool For CRPS-RSD Patients

"I was skeptical going in, but the author was very sensitive toward everyone's individual journey. The book never made me feel like my pain is "all in my head" or that there's any shame around need for meds. The book seems well researched, pulling from other well-known Neuroplasticity publications written by leading Neuroscientists in the field. Though, this information is much more accessible and digestible- boiling all the key concepts down into an easy conversational tone. I haven't listened to the exercises for 30 days yet, but I do have medical trauma that living with CRPS for 16 years has caused, and I do feel it's time to begin that healing process. My favorite parts of the book are the advice on Pacing and Self Care. Pacing can be illusive, but the author makes it clear, in bullet points. These will be perfect reminders for me going forward, taking better care of myself. Because it's written by a patient, she gives her favorite techniques specifically crafted for CRPS/RSD survivors.

I believe anyone with an intractable pain condition would benefit from reading this book"

-MaryMo - abodyofhope.wordpress.com

Table of Contents

A Message From The Author	*13*
The 4R's Neuroplastic Healing System	*16*
How To Use The Neuroplastic Healing System	*19*
CRPS ~ RSD	*22*
Module 2: Retraining The Brain For Pain Relief	*31*
Modern Discoveries In Brain Neuroplasticity	*31*
Module 3: Mind-Body Tools For Retraining	*38*
Module 4: Techniques To Retrain The Brain	*45*
The Pain Dial Technique	*55*
10 NLP Techniques To Reduce Pain	*56*
Module 5: Stress, Pain & The Limbic Brain	*61*
Module 6: Stress Control	*68*
Module 7: Breakthrough Therapy Technique	*83*
Module 8: Strategies To Take Back Your Life	*94*
Pacing And Goal Setting	*94*
Pain Friendly Diet Suggestions	*98*
Know Your Pain Triggers	*101*
Healthy Sleep	*103*
Self-Care	*105*
Module 9: Recordable Meditation Therapy Scripts	*109*
How To Record The Therapy Scripts	*109*
Module 10: Therapy Script #1 - For CRPS	*112*
Module 11: The Power Of Remembered Wellness	*137*
Module 12: Therapy Script- Remembered Wellness	*142*
Module 13: The 30-Day Plan	*151*
Resources	*153*

A Message From The Author

"God said to me, I am going to show you pain... and then you are going to help other people in pain because you understand it"
– Lady Gaga quote regarding her personal battle with Fibromyalgia

I posted this quote on my bedside table where I could see it every day. I knew one day that this pain, this thing I ferociously battled and then befriended would lead me down a path of helping other people in pain... become pain-free. – Carol Charland, Author & Wellness Coach

I understand the pain of CRPS- Complex Regional Pain Syndrome. I went nine years undiagnosed with CRPS, in horrific pain, allergic to narcotics with no relief. Like many people diagnosed with CRPS, it robbed me of who I was, my sense of purpose, a career that I loved and turned every aspect of my life upside-down.

My Story: I Am A Pain Patient With CRPS

I understand living a life of pain and the unique characteristics of CRPS. I know the frustration of going from one doctor to another searching for a correct diagnosis only to leave their office feeling more defeated than when I first stepped through their doorway. I know how it is to try one medication after another hoping it will work, only to have the treatment fail. Most of all, I know the feeling of being completely hopeless, that this "pain" will never end.

After nine years of life with CRPS, I was fortunate to receive the care of Dr Pradeep Chopra, MD an expert is CRPS. It was his treatment protocols that set me on the path of healing and my interest in neuroplasticity techniques and the limbic brain's role in being "stuck" in chronic pain. I have been in remission since 2017.

This program will teach you the same techniques I used to restore and maintain my level of wellness. I work at maintaining my state of remission every day. I use the same neural retraining techniques in this book to restore the limbic brain system, to control stress and calm the nervous system.

Written Specifically For CRPS

This program is unique and unlike any other you have previously used for pain relief. It is written specifically to address the unique symptoms and characteristics of CRPS. There are no other programs for CRPS like this one. The mind-body pain relieving techniques are proven successful.

As you begin to implement the program and practice the techniques, you will find some may have an immediate impact on reducing your pain and symptoms while others may take a bit longer to integrate.

Do not give up prematurely. Complete the program as instructed, repetition to create new neural pathways is key to your success. If you complete the program as instructed at the end of the 30-day period, you should notice a remarkable difference in your level of pain and your ability to self-manage pain. You may find the chronic pain once thought unchangeable may be reduced significantly or eliminated entirely. Continue using the program until you are able to reduce the pain and symptoms.

New Science. New Method. Amazing Results!

You will find the strategies in this book differ from the mainstream approach for the treatment of chronic pain and illness. It will teach you why other treatments failed to alleviate the pain and how a maladapted limbic brain keeps you "stuck" in pain and how to get "unstuck".

The techniques offered are for people living day-to-day with the task of finding opiate-free, effective pain relief while still trying to live a fulfilling life. The skills you will learn are practical and proven mind-body techniques that anyone at any age can easily learn.

I have seen people, and also experienced myself, that by using *Retrain Your Brain* methods, you can rise above chronic pain in an amazing way. When I used the tools of reframing to release the old stuck pain messages, it changed how I experienced CRPS pain, and my entire life changed for the better. I am now in a state of remission. You too can be more productive, can enjoy life once again and you may even find a new life purpose as I have in helping others suffering in pain and writing the *Retrain Your Brain* series of wellness books.

Neural retraining helped me to get my life back. It can help you too.

You will find that once you master the NLP Neurolinguistic Retraining Techniques found in this book, you can use them to achieve many other life goals that can help increase your overall joy and happiness in life.

I hope this will only be the start to a positive new beginning in life for you.
~ Carol

The 4R's Neuroplastic Healing System

Release~Reframe~Retrain~Restore Wellness

The 4R's Neuroplastic Healing System is designed to empower you take back control of your life from the grip of chronic pain. As you take an active role in your own healing process, it builds self-confidence in your ability to control pain.

It was out of my search for my own opiate-free pain relief, that I developed the *4R's Neuroplastic Healing System*. It reverses the stages the brain took when it created the condition by releasing the trauma from injury that was stored in the brain and created symptoms.

The 4R's Neuroplastic Healing System utilizes the latest neuroscience discoveries in brain neuroplasticity or how our brain can easily be retrained to "unlearn" old stuck behavior patterns once thought unchangeable… including chronic pain patterns stored in the brain.

This program is unique, unlike any other pain management program you may have used in the past. Unlike other generic pain relief programs, this program specifically addresses the unique characteristics, pain and symptoms of CRPS.

The 4R's Neuroplastic Healing System is based upon the latest discoveries in brain neuroplasticity and my professional training in neurolinguistics as a mind-body specialist since 1998. It is an immensely powerful healing system that can be used to achieve wellness goals that you once might have thought of as unobtainable. I used the system to conquer my own wellness issues and I continue to use this system to maintain my state of remission.

The program integrates the cognitive conscious thinking mind with the powerful subconscious mind that has the ability to influence the function of the body. Utilizing both the conscious and subconscious mind makes a powerful healing combination.

The 4R's Neuroplastic Healing System has four steps:
Release
Reframe
Retrain
Restore Wellness

Each of the four learning modules include step-by-step guides that teach you neural retraining techniques, which you can start using immediately. Each learning module builds upon the others to bring you back to a state of whole-person wellness.

Release: The 4 R's System teaches you a revolutionary technique developed by a physician who successfully treats PTSD, stress and trauma worldwide. It gets to the root cause of the limbic dysfunction immediately to release embedded "stuck" messages stored in the brain of injury, trauma and chronic pain.

Reframe: Reframing is a term used in psychology to change the way you think about something, thus changing how you experience it. Reframing has the power to change your mental perspectives and how you experience "things" in life, including how you experience pain and illness. It changes the internal image you hold of yourself switching from pain-mode to pain-free.

Retrain: The retraining step is designed to reboot and calm the nervous system. It creates new neuropathways for positive change. It builds stress-hardiness, resiliency and strength. You'll learn techniques that stop the "sick mode" cycle in the limbic brain. It teaches modern stress control that changes your emotional response to stress and activates your natural relaxation response so the limbic system is restored and your mind-body can heal.

Restore Wellness: This step is the return to a state of whole-person wellness. It gives you a toolbox of selfcare strategies to help you achieve whole-person wellness, health and happiness.

The 4'Rs Neuroplastic Healing System is your transformative path to healing that returns you to whole-person wellness mentally, emotionally, physically and spiritually

How To Use The Neuroplastic Healing System

This is a self-directed learning program you complete at your own pace. The success of the program requires a commitment from you to fully complete it and follow the instructions on a daily basis. You are the key to your success; you will get out of this course what you put into it.

You have all the resources you need to heal your mind and body. Like a flower planted in a garden you simply need the right conditions to bloom and flourish.

Key To Success:
· To obtain the best outcomes follow the instructions completely
· Don't give into negative thinking and self-doubt
· Don't listen to critics that make you doubt your body's ability to heal
· Don't quit.
· Trust the healing process
· Keep a written journal with photographs to document progress

This is your own personal healing journey. A method you chose because it resonated with a truth you hold deep within you. Don't quit prematurely. Your condition did not manifest overnight it took time to develop and healing is no different. Healing happens in its own time.

Most people respond to the neurolinguistic retraining techniques quickly and experience some noticeable changes in symptoms within ten - fourteen days. For some people the healing process may be more subtle and take longer. Be patient and be kind to yourself as you embark on this journey. Show yourself the same love and compassion you would to a loved one healing from illness.

A Commitment To Wellness

If a doctor handed you a prescription for a pill saying "take this pill for 30 days and you'll feel better" you would make the commitment to take the pill for 30 days without hesitating. Neuroplastic healing is similar, it requires a daily commitment to following instructions, performing the training techniques (generally only 30 minutes a day) and completing the full program.

Take Control Of Your Pain

I am not a professional writer, although it has always been my dream to write a book. I use an easy conversational style of writing, as if you were a client sitting in my therapy office. The book is designed to be an instructional tool to give you the tools you need to manage pain more effectively and get your life back from pain.

Pain-Patient Friendly

This book is pain-patient friendly. Pain patients experience unique learning issues like; brain-fog, memory, reading or problems focusing their attention. The book is a short, quick, easy to read book, concise and to the point. Instead of overwhelming you with medical terminology, it uses everyday terms anyone can understand. The chapters are set up as learning modules with step-by-step guides that walk you through the program and teach you pain relief techniques that you can start using immediately.

A 30-Day Program in Neural Retraining

This 30-day program is self-learning, it can be customized to address your unique needs. Simply read the book completely and follow the instructions. Use the daily plan at the end of the book to design your own selfcare pain management program that works best for you.

Medical Disclaimer

This book is not intended to diagnosis medical conditions. It is not meant to replace traditional medical care by your doctor but to compliment it. It is simply a self-help tool teaching mind-body techniques that empower you to manage your health better.

Note: Never use pain relief techniques for chest pain, heart or cardiac issues, abdominal pain or sudden onset of pain. These conditions can be serious, and you should seek immediate medical attention.

Please, check with your doctor before making changes to your diet, exercise or health care regimen.

CRPS ~ RSD

*Complex Regional Pain Syndrome also known as
Reflex Sympathetic Nerve Dystrophy*

The RSDSA Organization describes CRPS as a life altering pain syndrome. It is a neuroinflammatory syndrome with unique characteristics. If you are reading this book on CRPS, I am sure you are aware of the devasting effects CRPS has on people afflicted with it.

CRPS Complex Regional Pain Syndrome formerly known as RSD Reflex Sympathetic Nerve Dystrophy is most likely one of the most misdiagnosed conditions in modern medicine. CRPS patients are often times denied medical treatment for pain relief after being labeled as a drug seeker or psychotic by the unaware medical community. The opiate-crisis compounded this dilemma for CRPS patients when needed pain medications were abruptly lessened or taken away completely. CAM Complimentary-Alternative Medicine therapies have helped some pain patients fill the gap left by the opiate crisis.

It is rated the highest pain syndrome known to man on the McGill Pain Scale. The foretelling characteristic is severe disproportionate, unrelenting pain with unusual edema and skin discoloration that goes well past the time an injury would normally heal.

It generally effects a limb; arm, hand, leg or foot after an injury but can spread to other areas of the body. It can spread systemically involving all organ function over time. The primary symptoms of CRPS are complicated with a variety of secondary symptoms that can interfere with the entire function of the body.

The effected CRPS limb may be extremely sensitive to touch, so it is difficult to have clothing touch the skin or to wear shoes. There may be muscular contraction and loss of function of the limb.

People with CRPS face many challenges the most critical being that the medical community is unaware of this condition so people may go years without the correct diagnosis and effective pain relief treatment.

The Budapest Criteria

The Budapest Criteria is a guideline of symptom categories put forth by experts in the field of CRPS that has become the standard for diagnosis of the condition. There is no single test available to diagnose CRPS which only complicates the process of being diagnosed even more difficult.

Co-Morbid Conditions

There are co-morbid conditions associated with CRPS; Dysautonomia or POTS Postural Orthostatic Tachycardia Syndrome, MCAD: Mast Cell Activation Disorder, Gastroparesis, Central Sensitization Syndrome and Fibromyalgia further complicating diagnosis.

The symptoms of CRPS can vary from one person to the next. There are different types of CRPS; CRPS I and CRPS II. The symptoms may present as burning hot or Icy cold pain. CRPS generally appears after a trauma or injury like a fall, sprain, fracture or surgery (CRPS I) although there are cases after a simple blood-draw needle stick or bee-sting. Non-trauma onset is also possible. CRPS II has an onset after a known nerve injury.

CRPS is complex in nature to diagnose and treat. There is no known cure for CRPS as of yet but being diagnosed early onset and modern treatment has resulted in recorded instances of a remission-like states where people experience less pain and symptoms. Treatment is not a one-size fits all solution. What works for one person may not work for another in CRPS. Stepping out of the box by utilizing Complimentary-Alternative Medicine therapies like NLP Neurolinguistic Retraining Therapy in conjunction with traditional medical care can help you manage pain and symptoms.

CRPS: is found in women more than men. CRPS was formerly known as RSD Reflex Sympathetic Dystrophy and has previously been referred to by 25 other names only leading to more confusion by the medical community on what is CRPS. It is still considered a rare disease or low incidence condition. Most people go years undiagnosed it took over nine years for mine to be diagnosed.

The Limbic Brain Connection

CRPS effects the Limbic brain, which is our emotional-stress center. Overtime, the limbic brain becomes maladapted and "stuck" in the fight or flight stress response from the constant pain messaging being sent to the brain. Therapy to reset the Limbic Brain is recommended for any chronic pain syndrome.

You may find that you have secondary symptoms like, depression, mood swings, bursts of anger, brain fog and memory issues along with insomnia. Some people report headaches, unfounded anxiety or hypervigilance.

CRPS involves the Sympathetic and Para-sympathetic Nervous System which like a falling domino involves the Vagus Nerve, ANS Autonomic and Central Nervous System. Practicing regular stress control is key to keeping the nervous system(s) calm, which turns off the stress alarm (fight or flight response) in the Sympathetic Nervous System. By practicing stress control and natural relaxation methods on a daily basis you can reset a malfunctioning limbic system.

Become Your Own Health Advocate

When I was first diagnosed, the best advice given to me was to learn everything I could about CRPS to become my own health advocate. You may find that you have to become your own health advocate to survive the challenges of this disease, mainly due to the fact that your family practitioner is unaware of this condition and not up-to-date on the more modern CRPS treatments. A specialist proficient in the treatment of CRPS can save you years of pain and frustration searching for effective care.

Breakthrough Therapy Solution

This book offers you a breakthrough approach in selfcare pain management that treats the whole person and compliments your traditional medical care. It does not matter if you have had CRPS for one month or twenty years this pain relief program can help you. The goal is to make you an active participant in your own healing process and build self-confidence by giving you the tools to help control your pain levels.

The Budapest Criteria
A Guide For CRPS Diagnosis

All of the following criteria must be met to have a positive diagnosis of CRPS:

- Patient has continuing pain that is disproportionate to the injury
- Patient must have at least one sign in two or more of the categories below
- Patient reports at least one symptom in three of the categories below
- No other diagnosis can better explain the signs and symptoms

Categories
Sensory:
- Allodynia: pain elicited from things not normally painful like touch, clothing, temperature, somatic pressure or joint movement
- Hyperalgesia: hypersensitivity to pain, heightened pain from things not normally painful

Vasomotor:
- Difference in skin temperature
- Difference in skin color and appearance
- Skin color changes

Sudomotor:
- Changes in asymmetry in swelling
- Changes in asymmetry in sweating

Motor / Trophic:
- Decreased range of movement
- Motor symptoms; tremors, weakness, dystonia

Module 1: Introduction To Neuroplastic Healing

This program is meant to empower you to achieve your wellness goals by giving you the tools you need to successfully change old, outdated behavior patterns, including chronic pain patterns.

Modern Neuroscience: Past & Present

I always have had an interest in the power of the mind, and why we do what we do. When I was younger, I studied the works of Dale Carnegie and Norman Vincent Peale's power of positive thinking and using positive affirmations to affect personal life change. I later discovered NLP Neurolinguistics, which was founded in the 1970's by Richard Bandler and John Grinder. The foundation of Neurolinguistics is language usage and how our mind and brain perceive words. In the beginning, NLP Neurolinguistics Programming was primarily used in psychotherapy counseling and for personal success development. Today it is the innovator for modern Neuroscience discoveries in how we retrain the brain to effect personal change in our lives.

My interest in mind-body medicine came later in 1990's when it was labeled "new age" and there was not a lot of medical research and science to validate it.

Neuroscientist, Dr Candace Pert, MD changed the "new age" label with her Nobel Prize-winning discovery on how emotions are stored in the cells of the body and can direct body function. She wrote the books "*Molecules of Emotion*" and "*Your Body Is Your Subconscious Mind.*"

We now have multiple research studies in Neuroscience that proves that our thoughts, the words we speak, specific images we visualize and our emotions influence the chemistry and function of our mind and bodies.

Dr Pert's discovery catapulted medical research and public interest into the mind-body connection. Complimentary-alternative therapies became more accepted in mainstream medicine

We know from famous researchers like Dr Larry Dossey MD's books *"Healing Words; The Power of Prayer & The Practice of Medicine"* and *"Healing Beyond The Body: Medicine & The Infinite Reach of The Mind"* that the words we think and the words we speak are extremely powerful and have a way of directing the mind-brain-body even when we are unaware of it. Dr Dossey's work proves it is important to think and say the good words when we are in a healing phase. Our mind, brain and body are always listening. The sound of our own voice is very powerful.

Dr Dossey's research validates the use of saying positive affirmations in healing

New discoveries in the field of Neuroscience have proven that it is possible that by choosing specific "words and phrases" to address specific problems in our lives, we can rewire our brains to help break through behavioral blocks, solve problems and even heal our body of pain and illness. The work of Dr Norman Doidge MD's work in Neuroplasticity of the brain *"The Brains Way Of Healing"* that it is flexible, ever-changing and can be rewired to "unlearn" certain behavior patterns, including chronic pain and illness. Dr Doidge states in his book that he healed himself of an incurable condition using neural retraining to reset the brain.

Dr Doidge's research proves you now have the power to change old "stuck" behavior patterns once believed to be permanent or unchangeable

Dr Andrew Newberg MD, a Neuroscientist at Thomas Jefferson University and Mark Waldman a communication expert, collaborated on a book *"Words Can Change Your Brain."* In it, they write "a single word has the power to influence the expression of genes that regulate physical and emotional stress." When we use words filled with positivity like "love and peace" we can alter how our brain functions by increasing cognitive reasoning and strengthening areas in our frontal lobes, using positive words more often than negative ones can kickstart the motivational centers of the brain, propelling them into action.

Dr Newberg's discoveries goes much further than just the mind-body connection but in how the words we speak can actually change how the brain perceives reality or what is real from unreal. By holding a positive optimistic word or image in your mind, you stimulate frontal lobe activity. This area includes specific language centers that connect directly to the motor cortex responsible for moving you into action, and as research has shown, the longer you concentrate on positive words and images, the more you begin to affect other areas of the brain. Functions in the frontal lobe start to change, which changes your perception of yourself to a more positive perception of yourself and your abilities. He writes "Overtime the structure of your thalamus will also change in response to your conscious words, thoughts and feelings. We believe that the thalamic changes affect the way in which you perceive reality".

Dr Newberg's research validates the use of guided imagery or visualization as a way to influence how your body functions. As Dr Newberg's research has proven, an image of a juicy tart lemon can be as real to the subconscious mind as if you were holding a real lemon in your hand

You will learn an immensely powerful NLP technique called Role Modeling as one of the tools of the 4R's System. It uses Dr Newberg's discoveries in changing the internal image or perception of your state of wellness thus changing the physical function of your body.

The Birth Of Neural Retraining

Neurolinguistics and other alternative therapies are no longer considered "new age" phenomena it has become the foundation of new discoveries in neuroscience and the revolutionary new therapy called neural retraining.

Module 2: Retraining The Brain For Pain Relief

Modern Discoveries In Brain Neuroplasticity

Neuroscientists have proven that your brain is constantly being shaped and molded by life's everyday experiences. This one single scientific breakthrough in brain neuroplasticity has greatly changed the way we approach how we change unwanted behaviors and habits even ones thought to be unchangeable. Every thought you think and feeling you feel, strengthens the circuitry in your brain known as neural pathways.

Neural pathways are the foundation of your habits of thinking, feeling, and acting. They form what you believe to be true and why you do what you do. Using techniques such as Neurolinguistics to rewire or retrain the brain has the ability to transform our mind and bodies by mobilizing our thoughts and practicing new ways of thinking, acting and feeling.

Research into Neuroplastic healing has proven that we can mold our nerve cell network and literally change how our brains work by changing neuropathways

Forging New Neural Pathways For Change

I like to describe the intricate neural circuitry in the brain that forms neural pathways as a maze of interconnected walking paths or trails through the woods. The more you repeatedly travel the same trail over and over again, clearing away the debris or obstacles, the stronger and more permanently embedded the pathway becomes. When you repeatedly travel down these new neural pathways using new behaviors, the old unused path (or habits) begins to fade away. The most used path will become the strongest... it will become the default setting in the mind's master computer and be used first before a weaker less prominent one.

Like walking the same wooded trail, by repeatedly practicing the NLP pain relief techniques, you are paving new neural pathways that the brain will set as a "default path" automatically following the new behavior.

Repetition Is The Main Principle In Neuroplasticity Retraining

Every positive thought you think, words you speak reinforce the changes you desire and strengthens the brain's electrical grid or nerve circulatory known as neural pathways. Changing an old habit and forging a new neuropathway for positive change involves hundreds of millions of interwoven connections between nerve cells and nerve pathways. This pathway then becomes part of the mind-brain-body connection.

This new behavior or habit formation is dependent on repeatedly training our brain to create the new pathway. Some people see immediate results, for some it may take days or even weeks to notice a lessening of pain and symptoms, but do not quit the program. It can take up to 21 days for the brain to switch gears when changing habits. Follow the 30-day program instructions completely, repeatedly practice the techniques given to create new neural pathways and you will see the results you desire.

KEY: Following the 30-day program instructions is key to your success. Repeatedly doing the NLP pain relief techniques, listening to the audio recording and following a self-care regimen is key in reinforcing the new neuropathways that effect positive changes.

The Mind-Brain Body Connection

What we used to think of as the mind-body connection, we now know is actually the mind-brain-body connection. Your mind, brain and body are intricately connected together in a circuitry system of interwoven nerves and neural pathways that dictate behaviors; how you act, feel and think.

Activate Neurons And Open New Pathways

Positive feelings and emotions activate neurons and open the pathways. The more intense the positive feelings (joy and happiness) the more neurons are activated solidifying the new neural pathway. Feelings and emotions act as the glue that binds you to the new behavior or pathway.

Neural pathways are reinforced into habits through the repetition of intentionally thinking, feeling and acting full of emotion in the new chosen behavior.

Retraining The Brain For Pain Relief

The 4R's Neuroplastic Healing System rewires your brain from old, outdated behavior patterns. It helps change your pain levels by "releasing" the root cause of why your mind-brain-body ever developed it. Reversing the steps of how the brain creates a behavioral pattern or habit forges new neuropathways (behavior patterns), so you experience pain relief instead of the old "stuck" outdated chronic pain.

First of all, it does not matter if you have had chronic pain for one month or all of your life. This program will help you manage pain better. The subconscious mind has no time consciousness. It either knows you have pain, or you do not. You will be creating new neural pathways for pain-relief. Switching from pain mode to pain-free mode.

If you have tried different methods to relieve your pain and symptoms but have failed or even if you are hesitant in believing this program will work for you, if you follow this program completely, you will notice a significant change in how you experience chronic pain. You simply have to follow the program instructions completely; repeatedly practice NLP techniques as instructed and listen to the therapeutic recordable meditation script consistently.

The Subconscious Mind

This program is unlike any other; you will be using a part of your mind called the subconscious mind. There is the conscious and subconscious mind(s) that we use in retraining the brain. When you are awake, you use the alert conscious "common sense" mind to filter information. When you relax and sleep, the alert "filtered" mind relaxes, it is turned off and the subconscious mind becomes dominant.

You open the doorway to the subconscious mind when you relax, daydream and sleep. When you work with the subconscious mind you are tapping into the immensely powerful mind-brain-body connection where the mind instructs the body.

Learning more about the subconscious mind allows you to understand how this program works to help you achieve your wellness goals and can help you to create any new neural pathway to achieve any goal in life.

- You can access the subconscious mind through a state of relaxation, daydreaming, meditation, trance or sleep. So, when you use programs like this one, no deep trance state is needed… only relaxation.
- Like a computer, it has no mechanism to tell real from unreal. Words and images can be very real to the subconscious mind. Dr Andrew Newberg's research findings validate that using the

"right words" has the ability to change our perception of life and reality.
- It has no time consciousness
- It is dominant when you are relaxed or sleeping (your conscious mind is at rest)
- The language of the subconscious mind is pictures and symbols; it is how you talk to it and instruct it. Remember, it has no mechanism to tell real from unreal. This is why using guided imagery meditations in healing is so powerful.
- When you dream and see vivid images and symbols, it is the subconscious talking to you in its own language through pictures and symbols in your dream.
- We use NLP Neurolinguistics (words, phrases, metaphors) guided imagery meditations, visualization of symbols to instruct the subconscious mind to take action.
- We use these NLP techniques to tap into the mind-brain-body connection in order to instruct it and get the response we desire.
- Like a computer running on a software program, your subconscious mind acts on words, suggestions and images when told to do so.
- The subconscious mind is very literal, what you feed it… is what you get.
- NLP neurolinguistics is not hypnosis; no deep trance state is needed to be successful.

Rewire The Master Computer In Your Brain

The subconscious mind functions like a master computer; that runs off from a software program, it stores all information in your memory from the moment you were born, even though your conscious alert mind does not remember some things, the subconscious mind does remember. Like a database in a computer, it can be programmed to perform different functions (create behavior patterns and habits). It can run off from this outdated software program until you use the correct tools to delete it.

Behaviors patterns and habits come from a software package installed in this master computer in your brain a long time ago, most go back to when you were a child. If you feel your pain comes from an injury or trauma (psychological or physical trauma) this system can "re-program" the master computer in your subconscious mind releasing all of the old programming including pain and trauma.

In the past, when you have tried to change habits, your subconscious mind was still programmed to "pain-mode" the old way of thinking. No one ever deleted the old software program in the master computer.

Utilizing the powerful NLP Neuroscience techniques in the 4R's System, you are able to communicate directly with your subconscious mind to release and "delete" the old programming "stuck" in the subconscious mind all the way back to when the behavior pattern (chronic pain) first developed.

When the master computer in your subconscious mind replaces the old data software with healthy habits you desire, that is exactly what you will get. Your subconscious mind already knows how to do this. It holds in its memory what it is like to be pain-free, to be healthy, to be well.

Affirmation For Creating A Neural Pathway: *"I act, feel and think like a healthy happy, pain-free person would act, feel and think… as if, I have always been healthy, happy and pain free".*

Like a computer, when you change the "programming" in the subconscious mind, it is immediate. It simply acts on the new programming just like a computer would do when re-programmed to perform a different action. Most people notice an immediate change in behaviors and habits that gets stronger as you repeatedly practice the NLP Neurolinguistics techniques.

Oftentimes, in my therapy practice, I hear a client say, "I have no self-discipline to stick with things, I just don't have any willpower, will this still work for me?" The answer is yes, it will. Unlike other systems, this is based upon releasing outdated neural pathway programming and creating new neural paths re-programming the information in the subconscious mind.

We are simply undoing habit(s) that have been programmed in the master computer of your mind. It is as simple as clicking a "DELETE" key to delete an old software program on a computer and then installing new software.

KEY: Remember we are dealing with the subconscious mind, not the conscious waking mind. The subconscious does not work off from time or age. It does not even have a mechanism to tell it real from unreal. These NLP techniques simply reverse the stages of how the brain created the behavior pattern (chronic pain) and literally pushes the "delete key" on that outdated software program.

Module 3: Mind-Body Tools For Retraining

Medical Guided Imagery

Medical Guided Imagery is a mind-body tool used in retraining the brain. You have most likely heard of imagery or visualization work, much like daydreaming where you simply picture an image in your mind. Medical Guided Imagery uses medical terminology to tap into the mind-brain-body connection using symbols, images, and verbal suggestions to instruct the body to perform a certain behavior to enhance or change your health. It uses medical knowledge of how the body functions to instruct the mind-brain-body through symbols and verbal suggestions. For example, you may picture the symbol of a dial like the one used for the pain scale to represent your level of pain by manipulating the numbers on the dial turning the dial down to a lower number, you can help lower pain levels. Medical Guided Imagery can be an effective therapy for a wide variety of health conditions.

The medical terminology and symbols in the imagery are intertwined in a relaxing guided meditation with visions of a warm sandy beach to achieve your wellness goals. Think of Medical Imagery as a special code to talk to the body. It can be fun to create a Medical Guided Imagery script because you can easily encode a variety of symbolic messages that the mind-brain-body absorbs to change the internal function of the body. Although it is referred to as imagery, it uses all your senses and is experienced throughout the entire body not just in the mind. Medical Guided Imagery has been used in hospitals, medical facilities, and in private psychology practices for decades for a variety of health issues including for weight control, lessening the effects of chemotherapy for cancer patients, cardiac, diabetes, insomnia, anxiety, depression, pain management and even in surgical centers for pre-surgery anxiety and suggestions for rapid post-surgery healing. NLP Neurolinguistics and

Medical Guided Imagery is a powerful tool in mind-brain-body medicine used to communicate, instruct, and influence the function of the body

**Your subconscious mind is the doorway
to the mind-brain-body connection.
The language of the subconscious mind is symbols, so you communicate with the subconscious mind through imagery, pictures and symbols, linguistics, or word phrasing.
The subconscious has no mechanism to determine real from unreal… an image is real to it**

The subconscious mind never shuts off, it is always taking in information and storing it in memory, even when you are unaware of it. When you sleep, the subconscious is dominant and when you dream in pictures and symbols, it is talking to you. That is why using imagery is so effective, it is the language of the subconscious mind, it is how you communicate with it, and how you instruct the mind-brain-body to effect change.

Practice Exercise: What image would you use to influence change in your physical body and health? Get creative and write a short paragraph using medical imagery that will help reduce pain levels.

The Lemon Taste Test

Studies show with a functional MRI (an MRI of a working functioning brain) that the brain cannot differentiate between what is real or imagined. It has no mechanism to do that. For example, when we envision a tart juicy lemon, our taste buds automatically begin to pucker up to the sour taste of a lemon even though it is only a thought or picture of a lemon in our mind. In the same regard the memory of a favorite childhood treat can make us crave or salivate in anticipation of eating the food. It has been proven that images of a dry, dusty desert will make someone thirst for water. The subconscious mind is tapping into its memory databank to trigger an action; like pucker up for a lemon or thirst for water.

In the same way, when using a functional MRI, if you were to imagine or view a picture of a relaxing beach, your mind-body begins to relax naturally and automatically. It uses memory and life experiences to perceive a beach is a relaxing place. Your brainwaves will lower to an Alpha level when viewing the beach imagery which is the same as when someone meditates.

You really do not have to do anything, the subconscious mind does it all by itself, it knows what to do with the imagery by using memory, beliefs, and life experiences. If your surroundings are stressful, you can bring your mind to a place of calm by simply imagining a safe or relaxing place like the beach in your mind. The more you practice using a favorite place like a beach to relax and reduce stress, the more readily you will feel the results of the relaxation.

Practice Exercise: Lemon Taste Test

You can practice the Lemon Taste Test by simply taking in 3 deep breaths, exhaling fully, letting your muscles in your face, jaw and throat relax, relaxing your body fully. Then picture an image in your mind of a lemon, bright yellow, ripe, plump, and juicy lemon. See yourself carefully slicing the lemon with a knife and see the juice running on the knife and over your fingers. Breathe and relax again… Use all your senses, so you can smell the juice of the lemon, feel the juice run over your fingers. Now imagine taking a big bite out of the juicy ripe lemon. You can remember; you know the lemon is tart and sour. You pucker up, you can feel your taste buds pucker at the tart sourness of the lemon… just as if you really took a bite of the lemon. The Lemon Taste Test is an excellent practice for engaging the mind-brain-body connection through imagery.

Practice this technique until just the thought of a lemon triggers the "puckering" sensation in the body. You will be amazed at how easy it is to make this connection, how immediate and profound this connection can be.

KEY: Practicing the Lemon Taste Test helps to train your mind into quickly opening the door to the mind-brain-body connection. The more you practice this technique and ones like it, the more immediate and beneficial the mind-brain-body connection will be.

Practice Exercise: Practice this a few minutes each day to open the doorway to the mind-body connection.
- Write down your first impressions of practicing the Lemon Taste Test.
- What did you experience? Sour taste, puckering taste buds?
- Is the connection more profound, stronger, more immediate with practice?

Tapping Into The Mind-Brain-Body Connection

When you are in a relaxed state, the conscious alert mind relaxes (goes to sleep), opening the doorway to the deeper part of the mind- the subconscious and the mind-brain-body connection. The imagery of a warm sunny beach or any place you find relaxing can be used in the therapy script to relax the alert conscious mind, allowing the doorway to the deeper subconscious to open to the mind-brain-body connection.

There is a saying between mind-body behavioral specialist "Where the mind goes... the body will follow" what you think and believe... is what your body will experience.

Biofeedback & The Mind-Brain-Body Connection

Learning the Neurolinguistic techniques in this program is remarkably similar to using professional Biofeedback therapy found in most medical centers. Biofeedback teaches you how to use the power of your mind to control bodily functions. Biofeedback is a machine with sensors that attaches to your body. The feedback teaches you to change or control your body's reactions to things by changing your thoughts, emotions or behavior, for instance, biofeedback can pinpoint tense muscles that are causing headaches and then you make deliberate physical changes in your body, such as relaxing the muscles to reduce stress, relieve pain and it has even been used to help prevent child bedwetting in children. In the same respect, when using it for wellness or pain control, you can learn to control the functions of your body.

The ultimate goal is to learn how to use these mind-body techniques at home to achieve your pain relief goals and reduce stress. NLP Neural Retraining Therapy like Biofeedback is easy to learn and do, a typical biofeedback session lasts 30 to 60 minutes and most people see immediate results in habit change. Like Biofeedback the NLP Neurolinguistics techniques in this program will teach you how to control the function of your body and what you experience.

Positive Affirmations

Positive affirmations are a powerful tool to condition the mind to making new changes and reinforce the positive changes you have achieved. Modern neuroscience has proven that our voice is a powerful tool that can effect positive change. Positive affirmations when said on a regular basis work to reprogram the subconscious mind to your desired outcome.

The work of Dr Larry Dossey MD has proven that our thoughts, beliefs, and spoken words are immensely powerful and can influence your subconscious mind thus creating an outcome or a reality that you choose.

Say your affirmations daily; out-loud, in a self-assured, commanding tone with positive expectation

Adopt A New Mindset With Positive Affirmations

It is time to put your prior treatment failures behind you in the past where they belong. Do not let them rob you of your joy in life and new healthy mind and body. Adopt a new attitude of positive expectations with a "yes I can attitude".

Stop Self Criticisms & Negative Statements

It is important to remember that your subconscious mind is always listening and it believes what you say. The sound of your own voice is immensely powerful. Your subconscious mind responds immediately and without hesitation to your own voice. Stop negative self-talk, criticism and negative statements about yourself and start saying positive affirmations to reinforce wellness and your success.

Affirmations

- I act and feel free-of-pain and illness. As if I have always been healthy
- I have healthy habits and behaviors that support a healthy mind and body
- I am now enjoying a healthy fit body
- I can do this… and I do
- I love my body
- I have successfully released any old trauma (physical or mental) from the past… it is gone permanently
- I now have a healthy internal image of myself
- I now take good care of my body, my health and my well being
- I deserve to be healthy, happy and live free-of-pain or illness.
- I am happy, fulfilled and joyful every day

Practice Exercise: Choose a specific topic, then write your own affirmation

Module 4: Techniques To Retrain The Brain

Change Your Perspective... Change Your Behaviors

Changing your perspectives is everything. When you change how you see or think about something, you change your behaviors to coincide with the new thought process or perspective.

KEY: When you retrain the brain, you are not only changing your habits and behaviors but as Dr Andrew Newberg's research has proven internal functions of the body will automatically change as well.

The Power Of Changing Your Internal Self-Image

The way we see ourselves affects everything about us. You hold an internal self-image or perception about yourself that has been programmed into the subconscious mind's master computer. It is most likely an outdated image. This internal self-image is what guides your behaviors and habits. We use the Neurolinguistic technique of *Role Modeling* to change the internal image in the master computer and forge a new neural pathway.

Role Modeling: Reframe And Retrain The Brain

We've all at one time had role models or wished we could be like someone. We wished we could play sports like an Olympian or have the success of someone like Tony Robbins. In the subconscious mind, Role Modeling connects an image to what you want to achieve. It gives the subconscious mind a blueprint to imitate and follow.

The key to successful Role Modeling is using a very vivid imagination to envision yourself successful, achieving a goal, being who you want to be, filling the vision with positive feelings and emotion. Remember, dream big and make that vision big, bold and wonderful.

Role Modeling

Dr Herbert Benson, MD, founder of The Mind-Body Institute at Massachusetts General Hospital in Boston Massachusetts was one of the first pioneers in mind-body medicine to use the Role Modeling technique in healing. Dr Benson used the Role Modeling in a technique he called "Remembered Wellness" in his books *"The Relaxation Response"* and *"Timeless Healing"*.

Remembered Wellness

Dr Benson discovered that the subconscious mind holds the blueprint of a person's perfect health in its memory. When faced with chronic illness, pain or injury, the person can tap into the subconscious mind's blueprint of good health prior to any illness, pain or injury, and it could return to that state of good health helping the person to heal faster. Dr Benson has successfully used this NLP Neurolinguistic technique on people with diseases, chronic illnesses, and injuries.

The 4R's System uses Dr Benson's "Remembered Wellness" technique in Role Modeling to trigger the subconscious mind to return to the blueprint of good health. In the master computer of your subconscious mind, we will be creating a new internal self-image of you, healthier, happier and free of chronic pain using the Role Modeling technique. This will reframe and retrain the subconscious mind to a state of wellness.

Modeling is an amazingly effective Neurolinguistic technique for changing old perceptions stuck in the subconscious mind and achieving goals. You can use Role Modeling to achieve any goal, virtually for anything. Tony Robbins is a famous motivational speaker that teaches people how to be successful. He uses NLP techniques to reframe the person's perception of their ability to achieve success. Another example of Modeling is how Sports Performance therapists use it with Olympic Athletes where the athlete pictures themselves crossing the finish line, holding a gold medal, seeing their body perform at peak potential, believing they can be a gold medal winner. We will use it to change the inner image of yourself and your health held in the master computer of your subconscious mind.

The Recordable Meditation Therapy Script uses the Role Modeling technique. You will have the opportunity to picture yourself healthy, happier, free of pain or discomfort, as if you have always been free of pain and illness.

You will be using the Role Modeling technique to reframe the outdated self-image held in your subconscious mind of yourself and your level of health and wellness. Your subconscious mind will use the imagery in the Role Modeling technique to change the outdated self-image held in the master computer to a new image of someone who is healthy and completely free of health issues.

It is important when using Role Modeling that you use all your senses and make your new self-image very vivid, bold, strong and alive. You want to imagine yourself just as you genuinely want to be healthy, fit, active, happy, as if you have always been.

Role Modeling

Think of Role Modeling as planting fresh seeds in the garden of the mind, where new perspectives will grow, you will find that once you change your internal self-image, a new way of acting, feeling, and thinking occurs naturally.

Practice Exercise: Role Modeling- Part 1

Begin this exercise by taking in several deep cleansing breaths and relaxing your mind and body. Get in touch with the natural rhythm of your breath and settle into the comfort of your own body.

- Use your imagination and picture yourself as you would genuinely like to be... healthy, fit, happy and free of chronic pain or illness. As if you never experienced chronic pain or illness.
- Make the new image of yourself big and powerful, very vivid, as if you can feel it in every cell of your body.
- Make the colors bright and lively, see everything about yourself happy, well, successful and enjoying the highest potential of health and well-being that you can imagine.
- Evoke positive emotions feeling happy and well with the new image. You may want to hum a happy tune like the "Happy Birthday" song or "You are my sunshine" to evoke feelings of happiness.
- Picture this new image of yourself standing before you. Use your imagination and imagine you can simply step-into it... melt and merge with this new wonderful healthy self-image. From the top of your head to the tip of your toes... mentally, physically, emotionally and even spiritually, you are this person.
- Now reaffirm to yourself that this is who you are.

Imagine you are installing a new software program in the master computer of your mind. "This is who I am". Healed, healthy, pain-free and well. Repeat this exercise three times in quick succession taking several deep cleansing breaths in between the imagery.

Daily Practice

You will be using this Role Modeling technique daily. Each time you do this technique, the image should be more immediate, the feeling in your body changes, your mindset is happier. Use the same version of this self-image each time you practice this technique enhancing the image and the feeling of wellness each time.

KEY: Remember the research of Dr Andrew Newberg mentioned in the introduction. Pictures, images, thoughts, words can change our perception of reality and the internal function of our bodies.

The Swish Technique

Dr Richard Bandler a leading scientist in mind-body development, created a powerful technique called "The Swish Pattern" that literally retrains your brain to easily change from one pattern of behavior to another, by "breaking" the habit. It releases old, outdated habits and behavior patterns.

The Swish technique actually causes new neuropathways to form in the brain, it retrains the brain to easily accept a new realization or behavior. In regard to pain management, it is that of a person healthy, happy and free-of-pain and illness. Each time you practice the Role Modeling and Swish Technique together, you are retraining the brain to think and act differently. You are reframing in the mind to what you will personally experience. Think of the Swish Technique as deleting old software in the master computer of your mind.

Practice Exercise: The Swish Technique

This is a 2-part technique to release the "stuck" root causes of trauma (mental or physical), injury, chronic pain and illness. You will repeat the Swish Technique sequence for any trauma, injury, pain, symptom or habit you want to change. It incorporates the Role Modeling technique that you just used in the previous exercise.

- I want you to take one specific symptom that you want to change (like burning nerve pain, skin tender to touch, swelling, discoloration) and give it a symbol.
- Give this specific symptom any symbol that you choose, anything you want... whatever "symbol" pops into your head. (a block, a fire or flame, a hard rock, little gargoyle monster).
- Picture the symbol itself; feel it in your hand,
- Imagine you are holding the symbol in the palm of your hand.

Now put that image aside for a moment.

- Get in touch with the new self-image you created of yourself in the Role Modeling exercise. Bring back the happy, healthy image that you created.
- Make the new self-image excessively big; powerful, it gets bigger and bigger, bolder and bolder, enormously powerful and strong in your mind.
- Do this until it is enormously powerful and strong. (yes, you can picture yourself as powerful as wonder-woman or super-man)

Now put this image aside for a moment.

- Once again, picture the symbol (gargoyle, fire, flame block) of the symptom you want to change in your hand.
- I want you to imagine that the big strong healthy image of you... is smashing the symbol of the symptom into tiny pieces or simply let it fade away. It is overpowering it and breaking it up into little pieces. (If you use the image of a fire or flame, use a fire extinguisher to put the flame out. If you use a block, gently break it into pieces or fade it away, use an eraser to change the color, a softening gel to soften the area and for swelling shrink it in size).
- Begin to clap your hands together repeatedly strongly (3-5 times). Imagine you are literally changing the symbol in your hand, break it up into tiny pieces, fade it away, shrink it or erase it until it fades away to nothing.
- With the count of 3... make the pieces smaller and fade the image of the symbol away to nothing... Count: 1- it is getting smaller, 2- it's fading away to nothingness, 3- it is completely gone now. Permanently gone. You are free of that symptom at last.

- Brush your hands off... gone. You can imagine washing your hands with clean water to get the image off your hands.
- You are training your mind and body to release the "stuck" old behavior pattern.
- Acknowledge how wonderful it feels to set yourself free.
- Now, reaffirm the big, bold, strong image of yourself from the Role Modeling.

Repeat this exercise three (3) times in rapid succession. Then repeat it daily, you will know when you do not need to do this any longer as the symptom has changed.

KEY: You will use the Swish Technique to release stress, any trauma or injury and on each pain/ illness symptom you experience.

Burning neuropathy pain: use the symbol of a flame and water or a fire extinguisher to put out the flame

Pain area feels hard: use a rock as the symbol and break it up into tiny pieces or a fine ash. Soften the area.

Skin discoloration: Use an eraser to change the color of the body area back to normal, fading it away

Swelling: simply shrink the area to a smaller size, picture it getting smaller until back to normal

Stiffness of joint/limb: imagine a gel like softener, softening the area until its more flexible and softer.

Sub-Modalities & Anchors For Pain Relief

You will use these mini-exercises to tap into the power of your subconscious mind to assist you in changing your own mental perceptions of pain and illness.

Sub-modalities: We use NLP sub-modalities to reframe or change how you perceive pain. If you have burning, neuropathy pain and you are given the symbol of a fire extinguisher putting out a burning flame (your neuropathic "hot" pain). You may describe your pain as exceptionally large and all-consuming or hard and tough, you will use the appropriate sub-modalities to shrink it down in size, making it smaller until it fades and disappears. You can soften the area around the pain, loosening and relaxing it so it is not so hard. You may picture your swollen limb/hand/foot and you can reduce the swelling by using sub-modalities until it is back to normal size.

Anchors: NLP uses anchors which can be symbol images or gestures to trigger a mind-brain-body response. Much like in the Lemon Taste Test... your body will respond to an image it knows in memory.

A popular NLP anchor technique is when you press your thumb and forefinger together in an "okay sign," you can be given the suggestion that you will relax and be "okay" and free of anxiety when you make the "okay" sign.

Water is a convenient NLP Anchor to use, and it is used for relaxation in the Recordable Therapy Script. I have given you the NLP Anchor of water in the therapy script; when drinking water, picture it is flushing toxins, rejuvenating, refreshing, energizing your body. Water is a natural relaxant; when drinking the water, you relax, can control stress and anxiety. When you drink water, it is an automatic mind-brain-body response; you relax automatically into a state of calmness. Imagine the water is like taking a magical pill that helps calm and relax you, it soothes away stress and anxiety.

My favorite is the NLP technique called THE DASHBOARD. The dashboard is a powerful mind-brain-body control panel that has a variety of switches, gauges and dials with labels on them for sleep, pain relief, energy… you will set these dials to the perfect setting to program or instruct your mind-brain-body for a given response. For example, when you turn off a light switch at bedtime, you can program your mind-brain-body for peaceful sound sleep. For pain relief, you are turning the pain dial down from 10-Zero until your pain is completely faded away at zero.

Daily Visualizations

Your subconscious is going to be programmed to respond to these images… you can use them without listening to the entire mediation script by picturing the specific image you would like to use for example… take in a few deep breaths to relax then picture the pain dial in your mind and slowly turn the dial down to zero where you are free of pain. If you have a favorite NLP Sub-modality or Anchor that works best for you, record it on your mobile phone recorder so you can listen to it whenever you may need it to control pain.

The Pain Dial Technique

Each morning (and anytime throughout the day you need to) you will use the pain dial to lower your pain levels for the day.

- You will take 3 deep breaths… exhale and fully relax your mind and body.
- Picture in your mind the dashboard control center and the pain dial with numbers from 10-Zero
- Locate your level of pain on the dial (or you may simply start at the number 10) and begin to slowly turn the dial down with each exhale of your breath.
- With your breath, as you exhale you are turning the number down. Your body is relaxing, muscles are loosening, pain is subsiding with each exhale as you turn the dial down to a lower number…until it finally is fading away.
- Count down 10-9-8-7-6 breathe and relax with each number count 5-4-3-2-1-ZERO.
- You will repeat this up to 3 times until you have lowered your pain level to Zero.

The more you use this image, the more immediate and responsive your body will become to the imagery.

Remember, your body has no mechanism to tell it that this image is not the master control center for pain control. By using this imagery on a daily basis, you are creating a new neural pathway for pain control.

10 NLP Techniques To Reduce Pain

Learning these quick mind-body techniques is easy and fun to do. They are meant to be quick, easy to use anywhere techniques that retrain the brain for pain relief. With repeated use you may be amazed at the results.

Choose a few of your favorite techniques that resonate with you. These are meant to be techniques you practice daily and use as part of your daily plan. You will use these when you feel a pain flare-up is imminent to control pain levels. By practicing them daily (even on your good days when you are pain-free) you are creating strong neural pathways so that when you are in a pain flare-up, they will help you manage the pain.

People have become more aware of the mind-brain-body connection and the infinite possibilities of the mind to govern the body. Chronic pain sufferers can use these simple mental techniques to calm painful symptoms. In scientific studies, people who suffered severe injuries mentally envisioned more healthy oxygenated blood flow to the injured area and found that the wound healed faster. This is a great example of what the human mind-brain-body is capable of.

The following 10 mental techniques are to be used in conjunction with a state of relaxation. You can use deep cleansing breaths or The Inner Sanctuary Imagery to elicit the relaxation response in the mind and body. Combine the relaxation response with one of these techniques to occupy your mind. The more you practice these techniques the more immediate the response and the better you will become at facilitating your own pain relief.

1) **Mental Analgesia-** Get into a state of relaxation. (if you have a phobia of needles do not use this imagery) Imagine giving yourself a powerful injection of numbing anesthetic like Novocain. Use your imagination to picture a soothing icy blue color surrounding and

flowing to the painful regions. I like to use a soothing color like a cooling numbing blue. As the Novocain takes hold feel the numbing pain relief. This technique is effectively used in natural child-birthing and used in dental hypnosis for people allergic to anesthetics.

2) **Mental Analgesia By Transfer**-Get into a state of relaxation. Imagine a bottle of numbing anesthetic like a Novocain cream or gel, give it a soothing color, you can even put a pain relief name on the bottle of cream. Pour some on your fingers, feel the numbing sensation on your fingers. Then transfer the numbing sensation to the painful area, imagine spreading the colored cream or gel over the entire area. With each breath you exhale… Imagine the numbing sensation soaking in until the pain fades away. You can use this for achy joints or widespread pain. This technique is effectively used in natural child-birthing and used in dental hypnosis for people allergic to anesthetics. **You can also use this to reduce swelling in your joints or limbs. Imagine it is a special gel made to reduce swelling. Imagine the affected area being reduced in size, see it shrinking, getting smaller until you can picture it normal size once again. Practicing this technique regularly can reduce the swelling over time.

3) **Symbolic Imagery-** Get into a state of relaxation. This is an NLP Sub-modality technique where you manipulate the image to reduce pain. Amazingly, the mind usually sends you the perfect symbol image of an object to use for the pain or symptom you have. Here are some samples of imagery:
   a) Imagine your pain as an object (flame or fire) and then gradually reduce the hot burning pain sensation by manipulating the image. I like to use the image of a flame for the burning neuropathy sensation and then see a large fire truck or extinguisher putting out the flame. This is proven effective for neuropathy and widespread nerve pain.
   b) If pain is a large hard block; give the block a dark gray color and as you breath into the area, make the block smaller and smaller,

fade the color from dark gray to a soft white until it softens and disappears.

c) If you have skin tender to touch or tender trigger point spots, imagine breathing the warmth of your breath into the painful area; it loosens and softens, becomes more flexible, touchable, and the pain fades away with each exhale of your breath.

d) If you experience tight tense muscles like back or neck spasms; imagine filling the entire spinal column with warm golden sunbeams that flow out from the spine into the muscles, relaxing all the muscles with each exhale of breath.

e) If you have swollen joints, limbs, imagine "magical drains" on the ends of your fingers or toes… releasing the excess fluid from the swollen area until the joint or limb is back to normal size. Then use the Role Modeling technique to picture the joint or limb normal size on your body and simply imagine stepping into the normal healthy (joint or limb) body. You Can use Dr Herbert Benson's *Remembered Wellness* technique that we talked about earlier by imagining you are returning the swollen joint or limb back to its original size or "blueprint" before injury.

4) **Altered Focus**- Get into a state of relaxation. This technique demonstrates how powerful the mind truly is in altering sensations in the body. Focus your attention on any painful part of the body, then alter the sensation of pain by imagining it is something else. Place a different sensation on the pain, place a fun relaxing symbol or image like a smiley face on the painful area. This will distract the mind away from the pain sensation. The mind cannot handle two competing sensations or images at the same time. Make the new image bold, vivid, colorful and funny.

5) **Disassociation**- Get into a state of relaxation. This is exactly what it implies, you imagine placing the painful part of your body separate from yourself. So, the pain is no longer in the body. I like to put it in a box outside of my body and contain it. I put the pain in box

with a label on it, tape it up so it cannot escape and place it in a safe place but far away from my body.

6) **Sensory Splitting**-Get into a state of relaxation. Split or divide the pain sensations from one another. If you have burning nerve pain, separate it from the headache etc. Place each sensation in a separate container or box. Then imagine you can remove each container outside of the body and far away from the body.

7) **Mental Escape**- Use positive imagery to escape. You can use the Inner Sanctuary imagery in the meditation script or create a different favorite place for this technique. As you mentally escape, imagine you can also physically escape pain… you can imagine flying away, getting on a sailboat and sailing away from pain to escape the painful symptoms. Imagine being totally pain-free and stress-free as you escape. The relaxation response in the body helps lessen pain; the deeper you relax into the daydream the more powerful the pain relief.

8) **Counting**- Get into a state of relaxation. Counting is a good way to distract the mind. Count backwards from 100. As you exhale, lower the pain symptoms with each number as you count backwards. You can use the alphabet also, saying the letters of the alphabet backwards. This is a good technique for pain-induced insomnia. If you have difficulty falling asleep, try counting backwards and relaxing into a peaceful sleep with each number.

9) **Pain Movement-** Get into a state of relaxation. Move the pain from one place to another. I use this technique to move it out of my body. I use my breath to gather it up and breathe it out with each exhale. I use my breath to push it out into the air away from my body. This is an excellent technique for when you need quick pain relief, if you are at work, out with friends etc. you can use this without anyone really being aware of what you are doing- you are simply breathing and exhaling.

10) Distraction- Get into a state of relaxation. Find a favorite hobby, craft or a creative outlet to occupy your mind. Occupying and distracting the mind with something you enjoy doing can help slow down the pain messaging being sent to the brain. If you are absorbed in reading a good book or creating a painting the mind is occupied by this activity.

Some of these practice techniques and suggestions may seem silly to you, but that is your conscious mind's way of thinking. Remember, we are working with the deeper, more powerful part of your mind, the subconscious mind and it loves using it's language of pictures, images and symbols to communicate and instruct your body.

As an expert in neurolinguistic retraining and working with the subconscious mind, I can tell you that if you follow this program, practice the pain-relieving techniques on a daily basis, you will gain control over your pain and symptoms. Your subconscious mind will know what to do with these pictures, symbols and verbal suggestions that you are giving it for natural pain relief.

Module 5: Stress, Pain & The Limbic Brain

The Cycle Of Pain

Persistent Pain Triggers The Stress Response In The Mind & Body

Experiencing Constant Stress Causes The Malfunction Of The Limbic Brain

The Malfunction Of The Limbic Brain Creates A Vicious Cycle Of Pain & Illness Called "Sick Mode"
Where You Are Virtually Trapped In This Cycle Of Persistent Pain & Illness, Even After The Injury Has Healed

Understanding the role that chronic pain plays in triggering the stress response in your mind and body is important to the overall success of this program. It is the constant pain messaging sent to the brain that triggers the stress response commonly known as the "fight or flight" response. Being in a constant state of "fight or Flight" stress contributes to the malfunction of the limbic brain system creating a vicious cycle referred to as "sick mode".

The Limbic Brain

The limbic brain is known as the "feeling and reacting brain". Its structures are located in the midbrain region that include the amygdala, hypothalamus, hippocampus, and cingulate cortex. Part of the system holds emotional intelligence and your memory (memory through experiences creates habits and behavior patterns).

Its job is to keep you safe by activating your natural survival mechanisms. It is your mind and body's private security alarm system. The limbic system gathers information about your present circumstance or environment. It determines if there is a "threat" (including what you may be only a perceived threat) and signals your immune system, releases powerful brain hormones and activates your fight or flight sympathetic nervous system(s) to respond.

The limbic system can become maladapted by constant stress. It works well handling occasional stressors but not for long-term stress. It is part of our ancient brain and was not really designed to handle modern stress that most people face on a daily basis. Chronic pain where pain messages are constantly being sent to the brain triggers the body's natural "fight or flight" response and overtime can create a maladapted limbic system.

Because the limbic system is not designed for the overload of modern stress it can easily malfunction and get "stuck" in a destructive vicious cycle that can contribute to symptoms and major health conditions. People refer to this as the limbic loop. I refer to it as the limbic "sick mode" where the system is malfunctioning keeping the mind and body in a constant revved-up state of the "fight or flight" stress response.

Sick mode is when the limbic brain becomes maladapted from continuous stress, becomes stuck in a vicious cycle, it loses its strength and resiliency, making you vulnerable to chronic conditions

How Does "Sick Mode" Create Chronic Conditions?

The term "*sick mode*" refers to the malfunction of the limbic system due to an overload of chronic stress, which can come from both emotional or physical stress. The limbic brain becomes hypersensitized to stress and even minor stress events can be encoded in the brain just as if it were a major traumatic event.

The brain is then stuck in a continuous cycle of "*fight or flight*" stress response. The cycle of stress repeats itself over and over like a stuck recording in an audio player. The brain is overwhelmed creating sensory overload issues and Central Sensitization Syndrome of the brain.

Overtime the continuous stress response weakens the immune and nervous system making you more vulnerable to stress-related symptoms, autoimmune conditions, chronic conditions and can keep you stuck in the behavior pattern of chronic pain.

The Limbic Loop Or The Cycle of Sick Mode Continues Until You Take Steps To Stop It By Controlling Stress & Healing The Limbic System

The Limbic System Is Not Only Affected By Daily Stressors But By Other Factors As Well:

Chemicals: Including those found in household cleaning products, personal care items, plastics and foods.

Heavy Metals: Lead, mercury, cadmium

Environmental Toxin: Mold, algal blooms

Infections: Viruses, bacterial or fungal, including gut dysbiosis imbalance

Inflammatory Diet: foods that activate inflammation like high sugar, alcohol, gluten, dairy, food chemicals & preservatives

EMF: Electromagnetic field exposure

Trauma: PTSD, Past stressful life events including injury, trauma or abuse

The limbic brain is poorly suited to manage long-term stress that we find in our modern society. It becomes hypersensitized to stress treating even minor stress as if it were a major traumatic event

Constant exposure to stressors creates an adverse brain response that gets stuck in survival mode. You may become sensitive and begin reacting to things you wouldn't normally react to. Then the limbic system starts interpreting everything as a stressors or threat that needs to be handled. The brain literally becomes stuck in a vicious cycle or threat mode.

The Limbic Loop's Sick Mode

You may begin to feel anxious all the time for no known reason. Hypervigilance is common in this stage of sick mode. You may find it difficult to relax, to sleep, or even to sit still. As the stress is compounded by more and more stress to the mind and body, you may become highly reactive to "everything" especially to more stress, foods, scents, bright lights, noises, foods that you use to be able to eat without a food reaction, to touch and to environmental changes, even temperature changes.

Central Sensitization Pain Syndrome

Central Sensitization Syndrome is a condition of the nervous system(s) that is associated with the development and maintenance of chronic pain. When Central Sensitization occurs, the nervous system goes through a process called "fight or flight" or wind up. It lowers the threshold for what causes pain and subsequently comes to "maintain" pain even after the initial injury might have healed creating chronic long-term pain issues.

Central Sensitization involves both a heightened sensitivity to pain and hyperalgesia. It amplifies pain. Central Sensitization plays a role in many different chronic pain disorders including Fibromyalgia and CRPS. Central Sensitization involves specific changes to the nervous system where you may experience a hypersensitivity to noises, bright lights, touch, odors and experience brain sensory overload issues.

Dr Herbert Benson MD's research into the *Relaxation Response* has proven that regular practice of natural relaxation methods like using the relaxation response, guided imagery like the *Inner Sanctuary* meditation, mindfulness meditation and breathwork can all help calm and soothe the Sympathetic Nervous System shutting down the pain alarm that triggers the "fight or flight response" in the body.

Daily use of relaxation methods creates stress resiliency, making it less likely that life's little ups-and-downs trigger the stress response and if it is triggered it is more likely to quickly return to a normal state.

You can train the mind, brain and body for natural relaxation by using these therapies:

- Guided Imagery, The *Inner Sanctuary* Meditation
- Dr Herbert Benson MD's *Relaxation Response*
- Breathwork; breathing techniques to relax the mind and body
- Progressive Muscle Relaxation Technique
- Mindfulness Meditation
- My YouTube Channel of relaxing videos, music and nature sounds: **https://www.youtube.com/channel/UCKKjaTFc7WA5CAAkNwYSRog**

Stress-Reducing Technology:

- Biofeedback training (you can purchase hand-held units for home use)
- Light & Sound Mind Machines (Deep relaxation & stress relief)
- Brainwave Hemi-synch recordings (brainwave entrainment)
- Virtual Reality Stress Programs
- Some phone APPS for calming nature sounds.

When the limbic system is malfunctioning, the results are domino-like, adversely affecting the function of all the other body systems. You may find that one condition develops into others as the malfunctioning snowballs. Often times you will read of co-morbid conditions associated with a condition.

What Makes This Program Unique and Highly Effective

Not all retraining programs are the same. Yes, all programs state they retrain the brain, reset limbic function and restore wellness but how do they accomplish this?

This program is much different in its approach. It uses a revolutionary technique to release embedded stress in the brain that other programs do not use. The *Safe Haven* technique is scientifically proven successful in releasing stress and trauma that has been embedded in the brain. It releases stress and trauma from injury that you may be unaware of that was stored in the brain at the time of the stress.

The technique is a psychosensory modality that creates a neurochemical chain reaction in the brain called de-potentiation. It specifically releases stored stress and trauma in the brain. Thus, eliminating the root cause of "sick mode" and the ending the continuous "fight or flight" stress response in the body.

KEY: Effectively addressing the limbic loop's "sick mode" by treating encoded trauma in the brain and reducing stress overload can be the missing piece of the healing puzzle for people with chronic pain helping you to heal, feel better and return to living a happy life.

Now You Understand The Basics Of How A Maladapted Limbic Brain Can Cause Chronic Pain Conditions…

Let's Talk About How You Effectively Reverse It By Releasing Encoded Stress & Trauma From Injury In The Brain & Controlling Stress

Module 6: Stress Control

The Stress Response

Let's examine more closely how and why the stress response or fight or flight occurs. Our bodies come equipped with automatic responses to adjust to our environments that allow the body to function optimally. For example, the body tries to maintain its temperature even if the temperature varies greatly from hot to cold. When the body perceives physical danger, the body needs the fight or flight response to survive, for example if you step into the street and see a car rushing to you the stress response allows you to have the strength and energy needed to leap out of the way.

You'll experience a higher heart rate as the heart beats faster preparing the body for physical exertion, breathing becomes faster, muscles tense up getting ready for action, while digestion and other functions of the internal organs are actually slowed down.

The way the body behaves during the stress response is not meant to be normal everyday functioning it is intended to be used as a survival instinct to respond to danger. It is a built-in alarm system designed to protect you.

Whether the stress is physical or emotional the response in the mind and body are the same. The body releases adrenaline and other powerful hormones that prepares the body to actually fight or flee. Constant pain messaging being sent to the brain triggers the fight or flight response in the body, the same response as if you were under physical attack sending powerful hormones like adrenaline and cortisol into the bloodstream.

Overtime when the body repeatedly experiences the stress response but does not react physically in response, negative affects begin to appear.

When stress of any kind, physical or mental occurs often and overtime that is when it starts to interfere with the way the body is meant to function, and physical symptoms of stress appear.

Common Symptoms Of Stress

Stress can have a multitude of symptoms both physical and mental that interfere with many aspects of living a happy healthy life. You may feel anxious, tense and jittery, experience shaking and trembling, have digestive problems, change in appetite or a stomach acid reflux, headaches are common, and you may experience unexplained chronic pain from tense muscles in the neck and back, insomnia, and there are behavioral and emotional symptoms like isolating oneself, feelings of hopelessness, irritability and anger and depression are common symptoms of chronic stress over-load.

It is especially important for people with chronic pain to build coping skills that help you manage stressors and can help reduce the fight or flight effects of stress on the mind and body.

The number one strategy for managing stress is relaxation. Learning natural relaxation methods or the relaxation response is helpful because it reverses the stress response, often times immediately reducing stress over-load.

Drug-Free Relaxation

Relaxation is a very effective way to calm your mind and relax your body and relaxation techniques such as progressive muscle relaxation, visualization or medical guided imagery and mindfulness meditations are some of the best drug-free coping tools for stress management. When you feel more relaxed you will be able to think clearer be more productive and control stress better.

Identifying Your Stressors

Everyone's daily life naturally has some stress. As individuals we all have our own way of coping with stress. What may be stressful for one person may not be for another. The first step in any stress management program is to identify the stressors or what is causing your stress.

Modern Day Life

We all have times in our life that we become overwhelmed with the number of daily tasks to finish so we push to get things done, our minds are filled with anxiety and worry, we get depressed, irritable and moody, our bodies are tight and tense and filled with stress. Our job performance and careers, relationships, our physical and emotional well-being all suffer during these times. We may experience a variety of unexplained symptoms like digestive issues, insomnia, headaches, chronic aches and pains, high blood pressure and even cardiac symptoms all due to prolonged chronic stress.

For many people, the chronic stress has been going on for such a long period of time that they have become used to, it has become a part of our normal lifestyle. We can get so caught up in our daily stress-filled life, we simply lack joy and the pleasures that life has to offer. Unfortunately, it oftentimes takes some sort of health crisis or wake-up call for people to become aware of the actual amount of stress they live with on a daily basis.

Background Stress

Psychologists call the cumulative effects of adapting to more and more uncomfortable life circumstances *background stress* and chances are that unless you are already practiced at stress management and using methods of deep relaxation, you are experiencing it right now.

Our Alarm System

I like to use the analogy of a home alarm system to the how our body's stress response works. A home alarm system is designed to keep us safe by alerting us to the presence of danger by blaring loud noise or alarm, but our body's alarm system or stress response alerts us that something is wrong by creating changes in our neurochemistry or body function.

If you've ever experienced unexplained symptoms like knots in your stomach, acid reflux, tension in the head, tight tense muscles, sudden anger, panic attacks or the inability to focus   chances are your body was responding to the release of chemicals from stress overload.

Let's go back to the analogy of the home alarm, if the alarm is switched off altogether the home is exposed to continual danger without there being any way of your knowing about it until it is too late. It would be like walking through the home without any fear all along in the presence of a predator, while it might feel nice to be so relaxed and stress free, your body actually needs the alarm or stress response to alert you to danger.

The stress response also known as the fight or flight response prepares you to fight or to flee. We actually need the stress response but in the same regard need to learn to control it.

Resetting The Stress Response

We have a natural method of relieving stress within us but unfortunately for many of us the pace of modern life has led us to ignore our own natural stress control mechanism.

The main goal of any stress management program is to reset your internal stress response to a healthy "useful" system that you can manage on your own. We do this by balancing the stress response with its partner the relaxation response. The relaxation response activates your body's natural stress reduction system.

The Autonomic, Sympathetic & Parasympathetic Nervous System

Understanding how your natural stress control system works is key to activating the natural relaxation response in your body.

Your Autonomic Nervous System (ANS) keeps your heart beating regularly, your lungs breathing and ensures that every organ system in your body functions properly, without you having to do anything to manage it. It is made up of several other systems.

The Sympathetic Nervous System (SNS) which is the center for the stress response while the Parasympathetic Nervous System (PNS) is the center of the relaxation response which is meant to balance the SNS. These two systems are meant to work harmoniously together with the Autonomic system.

Imagine yourself going for a walk on a nice sunny day and suddenly a vicious looking dog appears and is coming right toward you. What do you do? Do you turn and run or stay to defend yourself?

It is the job of the Sympathetic Nervous System that governs the stress response (fight or flight response) to flood your system with powerful hormones like adrenaline to pump extra blood and oxygen to your limbs so that you can run away more quickly or fight with more strength. The SNS plays a vital role in our survival however when left unchecked all the powerful hormones like adrenaline take a toll on your health.

After the situation with the vicious dog is resolved and you are safe, it is the job of the Parasympathetic Nervous System known as the "rest and digest" system (the relaxation response) that brings your mind and body back to a state of normal calm or relaxation. It is designed to bring balance back to the Sympathetic System. The Parasympathetic Nervous System is responsible for the relaxation response, it is your body's natural balance to the stress response. This is your built-in internal survival mechanism, designed to protect you and then return you to a normal state of rest.

You experience many types of stress on an average day, driving to work stuck in a traffic jam, argument with a family member, coworker or friend, an unexpected bill arrives in the mail, or the kids make a mess in the house before relatives arrive. These little things may not consciously seem like threats to you, but your nervous system cannot differentiate between a physical threat to your body and a mental or emotional threat.

"It is not the event but rather our interpretation of it, that causes our emotional reaction"
- Dr Hans Selye

Key: Remember controlling stress is a mind game, it is mostly about perception. What you "perceive" as a threat becomes a stressor whether it is truly a threat or not. If your boss criticizes your work, your mind responds to the situation with the stress response, it produces powerful hormones that flood the bloodstream with the same chemicals produced if you were under physical attack.

The Relaxation Response

Dr Herbert Benson MD's research into the *Relaxation Response* has proven that regular practice of natural relaxation methods like using the relaxation response, guided imagery like the *Inner Sanctuary* meditation, mindfulness meditation and breathwork can all help calm and soothe the

Sympathetic Nervous System shutting down the alarm that triggers the "fight or flight response" in the body.

Daily use of relaxation methods resets the limbic system by creating stress resiliency, making it less likely that life's little ups-and-downs trigger the stress response and if it is triggered it is more likely to quickly return to a normal state.

Finding Inner Peace

What does inner peace mean to you? Everyone has an idea in their mind of what they think inner peace is. You want to be able to create this feeling of inner peace in your life without it being dependent upon other things like how a certain person acts, how your job is going or how certain life issues turn out. You can achieve this by simply changing your perspective, focusing on the positive rather than the negative.

Inner peace comes from within you... not from the things on the outside of you. The goal is for you to take inner peace and bring it to your outside world. You have the ability to do this by using the neurolinguistic techniques in this program.

You have the ability to change your perspectives on how you experience life. One of the ways to bring inner peace is to calm the mind... and calm the body.

Become mindful- You can create balance and stability by calming down and taking a few moments to think before you act.

Most people get so busy with their lives they forget to pause and check-in. Many of us engage in continuous motion, going from one thing to the next and the next without stopping. It is important to pause and take a mental break if you want to feel calm, stable, and balanced.

Stop and pause throughout the day, have a mindfulness moment, focus on what you are doing, change your perspective, quietly experience relaxation, a quiet mind brings a different level of awareness and inner peace. It can bring your emotions into a state of peace and quiet that becomes inner peace.

Steps For Quick Relaxation To Calm the Mind And Body

Natural relaxation methods elicit the relaxation response, which counteracts the fight or flight stress response in the body. It helps naturally calm your mind and body. Some key symptoms of anxiety include tight tense muscles, shallow rapid breathing, worried thoughts and shaking. Natural relaxation methods target anxiety and its symptoms.

Breathe! Focus on breathing, calming your breathing is key to being calm and relaxed. Use a mantra or phrase while doing the breathing exercise to connect your mind and body with calmness. "I am calm and relaxed"

Take 3 deep cleansing breaths… inhale through your nose… exhale through your mouth… just as if you are blowing out a candle… blow out all the air like a big sigh of relief… imagine calming your mind and body with each breathe.

…as you inhale focus on slowing down, you're breathing to a calm rhythm… exhale fully all the way down into your abdomen… releasing all of the air… continue to breathe slowly and calmly rhythmically.

You realize that you are getting all the oxygen you need, realize that your only job right now is to keep yourself as calm and comfortable as possible until the feeling of anxiety passes… fighting against the anxiety only makes it stronger so right now except that you are feeling anxious… and focus on calming your thoughts to relieve the anxiety.

Progressive Muscle Relaxation

Finally, focus on how to relieve anxiety by relaxing the physical body with the progressive muscle relaxation technique. It can help relax the physical body by releasing the tension held in muscles.

Practice Exercise: Get in a comfortable position and into a mental state of relaxation by taking several deep cleansing breaths. You begin by relaxing one area of the body to the next. Focus your attention at the top of your head. Imagine a warm wave of relaxation (give it a beautiful soothing color) and as you exhale your breath move it from the top pf the head to the face, the jaw, the throat. As you move the wave of relaxation all the muscles in the body release stress and tension, soften and relax. Keep moving the relaxation down your shoulders and arms, down your back and spine, down your chest and abdomen. Then move it down your legs to your feet and toes.

The key to successfully using progressive relaxation is to actually feel the tension (pain or discomfort) in the area soften, release and relax. Keep repeating the cycle from top of the head down to the toes until you feel muscles completely relax. The more you practice this technique the more automatic and immediate it becomes.

You can combine imagery with this technique. You can use color by visualizing a soothing calming color as a wave of relaxation flowing from one area of the body to the next.

The Inner Sanctuary ~ Relaxation & Natural Stress Control

You will be creating your own *Inner Sanctuary* to mentally escape, relax naturally and reduce chronic pain and stress. When you practice natural relaxation methods on a regular basis, you are building a neural pathway of calm resiliency and inner strength. You can use this technique to help you sleep better and during times of anxiety to calm the nervous system.

You should practice the *Inner Sanctuary* natural relaxation method regularly to control the stress response in the body. I use the image of the beach in the Recordable Guided Imagery Script, so your subconscious mind automatically connects the image with relaxation. The Inner Sanctuary becomes your favorite place for escaping stress and a place you can go to relax. Using natural relaxation methods re-sets the relaxation response automatically in the body, bringing balance and harmony back to the stress response.

The practice exercise uses Guided Imagery and the Progressive Relaxation Technique to relax all the muscles from the top of the head to the tip of the toes.

Practice Exercise: Create Your Own Inner Sanctuary

You can use the beach imagery from the Recordable Meditation Script found at the end of this book to create your own *Inner Sanctuary* or create your own imagery script of a favorite place; perhaps a serene lake, a cozy mountain cabin or a beautiful spring garden full of flowers.

Whatever scenery you create for your *Inner Sanctuary*, always envision yourself relaxed, healthy, happy and well in this special place. Use all of your senses to place yourself there. Add joyful emotions, soothing calmness to the imagery. You can add the Progressive Muscle Relaxation technique and positive affirmations to this special place you go to rest, relax and escape stress and pain.

You create your own private escape. If you feel stressed, overwhelmed, having a difficult day… you will immediately use this technique to relax the mind and body.

If you practice this technique daily, you should feel the results quite immediately, as soon as you go to your Inner Sanctuary. You will be amazed at how quickly the "Inner Sanctuary" appears in your mind and you feel relaxation filling your mind-brain-body. By practicing this technique, you are programming your mind-brain-body for instant relaxation.

Helpful Tips For Managing Stress

LIFESTYLE: Lifestyle changes like exercise, sleep, diet and weight management, stop smoking and selfcare can help lessen the effects of stress and anxiety. **NOTE:** I offer stress management, smoking cessation and weight management programs that use neural retraining in my private practice. To learn more about these wellness programs visit my website.

CAM: Combining CAM- Complimentary-Alternative Medicine with your traditional medical care can help put you in control of stress, panic attacks, anxiety and fears. Natural relaxation methods are very effective in combating fight-or-flight anxiety.

Finding ways to calm the "fight or flight" response that is triggered by stress response is key. Practicing natural relaxation techniques like the ones you will find in this program can help you develop the ability to cope more effectively with stress. In this program you will learn a variety of mind-body techniques like The Relaxation Response by Dr Herbert Benson of The Harvard Mind-Body Institute in Massachusetts, progressive muscle relaxation and NLP Neurolinguistic Medical Guided Imagery techniques to help you relax naturally, relieve stress, anxiety and fear.

Some other CAM Complementary Alternative Medicine therapies you may want to consider would be Mindfulness mediation, yoga or Tai chi, guided self-hypnosis, acupuncture, massage and energy healing like EFT or Reiki.

EXERCISE: Regular exercise can help strengthen the body, boost the immune system and boost your moods by releasing Endorphins. Exercise may even help you sleep better at night. Start out slow, pace yourself and avoid over exercising. Remember to always check with your doctor(s) before beginning any new exercise or health regimen.

REST: Get a good night's sleep. Being well-rested can help you cope with stress better. Setting a sleep routine with regular sleep and wake times, having a quiet dark room in a soothing environment can help. Avoid stimulants like watching TV, being on the phone or computer in bed and avoid drinking caffeine late at night. All these can help promote a deeper more peaceful sleep.

NUTRITION: Eating healthy is just good healthcare, it is particularly important if you are under chronic stress. Avoid caffeine and alcohol which can trigger anxiety. You may want to try "clean eating" cut out fast food, canned or boxed foods loaded with preservatives, and eat fresh organic fruit, vegetables, poultry or fish. Please remember to check with your medical doctor before starting any new diet or health regimen.

 NOTE: I offer weight management programs in my private practice that use neural retraining techniques to help eliminate unhealthy eating habits, lose weight and stay on a healthy diet. Please visit my website for more details on *"The Mind-Body Weight Loss System"*.

SUPPORT SYSTEM: Finding a support system that understands what you are experiencing, where you can talk about worries and concerns can help. Professional counseling or a group with other people suffering with similar issues may help you. Sometimes just the act of talking out-loud about an issue instead of keeping fears bottled up inside can help resolve it.

TOBACCO: Cut out nicotine and tobacco products. I know most smokers use cigarettes as a relaxant but in truth the nicotine in cigarettes trigger adrenaline which in turn triggers the fight-or-flight response in the body. Smoking fills your body with harmful toxins that can elevate pain levels.

NOTE: I offer smoking cessation in my private practice. I use modern neural retraining to help you become a non-smoker. You can learn more about my *"Successfully Stop Smoking in 14-Days"* program on my website.

SELF CARE: Selfcare is healthcare… it is you taking good care of yourself; mentally, physical and spiritually. Creating your own Self-Care regimen can help ensure that you follow through on a regular basis. Set time aside to do something you love doing, makes you feel good about yourself and is soothing to you. Selfcare can be many things, perhaps it's a creative outlet like crafts or hobbies, keeping a journal, a mental distraction where you can escape stress for a while. It's okay to pamper yourself. Some people mistake self-care for being egotistical only taking care of yourself or think of it as a luxury, when in actuality it is an essential part of our overall wellbeing.

Module 7: Breakthrough Therapy Technique

There are many reports of the onset of CRPS and other pain syndromes like Fibromyalgia following injury and trauma. The trauma of the injury is encoded or stored in the brain creating chronic pain conditions.

The Havening Technique

The Havening Technique is a powerful technique used to release stress and the trauma of injury stored in the brain.

> *"The mind is released from darkness once we shine the light of a safe haven through touch"*
> *- Dr Ronald Ruden, MD*

The Havening Technique (HT) is a new and revolutionary way to heal emotional disorders associated with stress, injury and trauma. Disorders like depression, post-covid stress, PTSD, fear or phobia, anxiety, hypervigilance, grief, anger, resentment, chronic pain and the physical illnesses oftentimes associated with these disorders such as insomnia, digestive issues and unexplained chronic pain.

Havening was developed by two brothers Dr Ronald Ruden, MD and Dr Steve Ruden, DDS. Dr. Ronald Ruden studied how the brain encodes (stores) traumatic memory and how it acts upon the stored memory. The Havening Technique is a way to safely remove the negative affect of trauma on the mind and body without the person having to re-live the traumatic event.

Many people find it difficult to talk about traumatic events, with the Havening Technique there is no need to re-live or talk about the event. It may be difficult for some people to pinpoint specific emotions and for others there may be a sense of shame or guilt associated with an event that stops them from talking about the trauma to anyone. HT can help you release encoded (stored) trauma in a safe, gentle manner without talking about the event. It can be used in conjunction with any therapy, it compliments both traditional cognitive talk therapy and complementary-alternative methods of healing.

How Havening Works To Clear Trauma Symptoms

Havening sets off a neuro-electro chemical chain reaction in the brain which leads to a process called depotentiation or a dismantling of the stored trauma memory. Havening is unlike any other healing method; it deals with specific symptoms associated with a traumatic event encoded in the brain.

Havening will seek out the emotion associated with a specific encoded event that causes a specific symptom (pain, depression, PTSD, fear, anxiety, fatigue) and dismantles the link between them. Once the encoded event is found and dismantled the individual experiences relief of all symptoms. It can be a symptom associated with several events that is dismantled in one Havening therapy session, thus releasing trauma symptoms from several events not just one. Havening has the power to release the root cause of the symptom completely and fully.

Remarkably after the Havening Technique has been completed to dismantle the traumatic memory there is no emotional connection to the event. You may or may not remember the event, but the traumatic response to the event is no longer present. Recall of the event no longer triggers emotional or physical symptoms like pain.

The Process of Depotentiation

The healing process that takes place with Havening is called depotentiation which breaks the emotional links associated with a specific traumatic event. The event can be completely depotentiated (**dismantled**) without talking about the details. There is no pressure to talk or re-live painful events when using HT.

How To Use The Havening Technique For Chronic Pain, CRPS & Fibromyalgia

The Havening Technique can be used on "events" that caused your injury and the onset of the CRPS or chronic pain. For example; If you fell and fractured your wrist and later developed CRPS in the injured wrist, use the Havening Technique on the injury causing event and then another session of Havening on the onset and symptoms of CRPS pain.

The Science Behind The Havening Technique

For the non-medical layperson, the scientific explanation of Havening is lengthy and may be difficult to understand. You don't need to understand the science behind Havening in order to perform the technique and reap the many benefits.

The following web links direct you to the scientific explanation (just in case you need that) and videos from Dr Ruden's website on how to perform the Havening technique. The technique has developed many variations and is now used for many other issues not just trauma.

Learn more about the scientific process of Havening: Havening: a complete scientific explanation of the processes that take place in the brain in how it encodes stressful or traumatic events and how the Havening Technique releases the encoded memory through a neuro-chemical chain reaction called depotentiation.

https://www.sciencedirect.com/science/article/pii/S1550830718301848

Learn More about Dr Ronald Ruden Founder of The Havening Technique and view videos demonstrating the technique
Dr Ronald Ruden MD

www.havening.org

You will find many variations of the Havening Technique that you may choose from. The videos on Dr Ruden's website and his YouTube Channel give you samples of the various techniques.

A Safe Haven: The Havening Touch Technique (HTT)

The Havening Technique uses the simple touch of your own hands in this amazing self-care treatment. Soothing gentle touch is applied to the arms, hands, and face. Through touch receptors in your skin HT produces special brain waves called delta waves which act directly on receptors in the brain where stress and trauma is encoded (stored).

The Power Of Human Touch

Dr Stephen Ruden discovered repeated touch to parts of the body produces delta waves when combined with specific lateral eye movements (similarly used in EMDR therapy) and visualizations of something pleasant have a predictable effect on encoded feelings. The delta waves elicited by human touch are what enable a mother to comfort her baby and is hardwired in the brain of every person.

Havening combines these deeply-seeded patterns of reassurance and comfort from human touch with sequences that breakdown unhappy feelings stored in the brain. This process elicits a rapid response, with just a few minutes of using the Havening technique, you should feel stressful emotions dissipate and experience calm relaxation.

A Psychosensory Therapy

Havening Touch is considered to be a psychosensory therapy in the same category with EMDR (eye movement desensitization reprocessing), TFT (thought field tapping) and EFT (emotional freedom technique).

Psychosensory therapy is a form of therapeutic treatment that uses sensory stimuli (touch, smell, sight, hearing) to affect psychological and emotional well-being. It has roots in traditional Chinese medicine and with the latest neuroscience discovery in brain neuroplasticity it has found its place in neural retraining programs with amazing results.

According to the *American Psychiatric Association* (Journal 2016), psychosensory therapies are effective for treating mood disorders, general anxiety disorders, PTSD and depression. It also can release the injury and trauma encoded in the brain that may be the catalyst for chronic pain syndromes. The pain messaging from an injury or trauma being sent to the brain simply gets "stuck" constantly repeating itself well after the time the injury has healed. The Havening Technique is used to release the memory "stuck" in the brain of injury or trauma thus releasing the symptom of constant pain.

All of these psychosensory methods are mind-body interventions used to make changes to encoded or stored emotion and thought patterns stored in the brain. Most of the time people are unaware that the episode was ever encoded and stored in the brain.

Havening is a self-treatment. You can self-haven or have someone else do the technique with you

A Clinical Study On The Havening Technique

A Study on the Havening Technique was published September of 2020 in the *Journal of Psychophysiology*. This clinical trial examined the impact of Havening Techniques on trauma responses in 125 participants. The study states there is evidence to the effectiveness of the Havening Technique creating sustainable long-term decrease in biological markers of stress and trauma while encouraging psycho-physiological resilience. Havening increases the levels of serotonin which can disrupt the consolidation of the link between the traumatic memory of the event and the distress that it causes.

The Havening process works surprisingly fast, often one session brings soothing calm and relief

Use For:

- For chronic pain issues; unhealed injuries,
- After a stressful or traumatic event (so event is not encoded)
- To calm "fight or flight response in the nervous system
- To self-soothe, to reduce anxiety and calm yourself
- For insomnia, calm a racing mind to sleep better
- Stop worrying, stop renumerating or over-thinking events
- To reset the limbic brain system; stop "sick mode"

It Has Many Benefits:

- Clears a wide range of issues both emotional and physical
- No need to re-live or talk about the event
- Combines with other therapies
- Can clear symptoms associated with several events simultaneously in one session
- Permanent clearing of emotional connections to an event

It Can Relieve:

Anxiety
Depression
Fear and Phobias
Grief
PTSD
Shock Or Trauma
Anger
Resentment
Worry and Renumerating
Chronic Pain Symptoms
Insomnia

The Havening Technique

Practice Exercise: The Havening Technique

Think of a specific event or stuck emotional block that you want to use the Havening Technique on. (the injury event that was the onset of the pain). Do not re-live it, simply use your memory to recall what it feels like in the body. Notice how much discomfort, anger, sadness, fear, anxiety that you feel so you can rate it on a scale of 0-10

Rate your Subjective Unit of Distress (SUD): From zero to 10. With Zero being no emotions at all and 10 being extreme distress when you think of the event. Rating the distress gives you a starting point, as you perform the technique you will be able to compare the distress you feel after performing the technique and how quickly the rating decreases.

The Eye Movement: Keep your head straight and slowly move your eyes laterally from left to right and back to the left. Do this eye movement repeatedly as you do each step of the Havening Technique to the arms, hands and face. This specific eye movement produces delta waves in the brain. Delta waves are ideal for reprogramming the mind, brain and body and used specifically for neural retraining.

Clear Your Mind: Think or visualize something pleasant. You can imagine walking along a relaxing beach or magnificent garden pathway. If you are not fond of visualization, you can hum a happy tune like the happy birthday song. It is anything pleasant that emits a sense of joy, happiness and is calming. This step is not only meant as a distraction to the mind but is used to elicit brain chemicals connected to feelings of happiness that change the way the brain processes our thoughts and feelings.

Start Havening - Arm Caress: Clear your mind, breathe, relax and start the Havening Technique by crossing your arms in front of your chest, place your left hand on the right shoulder, your right hand on the left shoulder. Simultaneously with both hands, rub arms downward with a soothing caress to your elbows and then back up to the shoulders as you caress the arms think of something pleasant like a walk on the beach, you can even hum a happy song like the happy birthday song if you like. While caressing the arms and thinking of something pleasant, you will use the side-to-side eye movement described above. Repeat this sequence of the downward stroke of the arms 20 times.

Hand Caress: Continue Havening by rubbing the palms of your hands together in a back-and-forth continual motion. Think of something pleasant and move your eyes from side-to-side. Repeat the back-and-forth movement 20 times.

Face Caress: Continue to apply Havening by gently rubbing your face with both hands. Across the forehead, over the eyelids, across cheeks. You may get an intuitive impulse to direct your hands to a specific area to caress. Think of something pleasant and move your eyes side-to-side. Repeatedly caress the face 20 times.

Affirmation: When you finish Havening, simply grasp your shoulders as if you are hugging yourself. Say a positive affirmation or word (I am pain-free, I am safe. I feel happy. I am healed. I feel strong)

Finally, Rate Your SUD: Rate your SUD from Zero – 10. Has it lessened from when you first started the technique? Continue the Havening Technique until your SUD is zero.

Practice Exercise: Make a list of events, symptoms and issues to use for Havening

While Havening and caressing the arms, hands and face, intuitively you may be prompted to caress your heart, your stomach or another part of the body. I always use the Havening Touch on this area as well. You may be amazed that you are prompted to caress the stomach and you have digestive symptoms or unexplained pain in the area you are prompted to caress. We know from the work of Neuroscientist, Dr Candace Pert MD that the cells in our body store emotions. You may be pleasantly surprised how an area of the body once tight, and tense will completely relax using the Havening Touch sequence.

As you perform the Havening Technique or any psychosensory modality, other emotions, words or events may come to the surface. You may feel angry, sad, resentment, guilt, grief or loss, depressed, unloved, unworthy and others. You will want to Haven this feeling, word or event that surfaced as part of the therapy sequence to release the encoded emotions and trauma associated with this specific event. Use the SUD rating on each emotion or word that surface.

Important Note: You can begin the process slowly by using Havening on a minor issue; perhaps you are feeling stress from work today, frustration or sadness before you apply it for any major traumatic or stressful events.

Practice Exercise:
Watch Dr Ruden's instructional video demonstrating the technique on his website (www.havening.org) and self-apply the Havening Technique as you watch his video.

Set Yourself Free With The Havening Technique

The Havening Technique heals trauma, but it also has the power to set you free from habitual negative thinking, lack of self-confidence and poor self-esteem that has previously sabotaged your personal goals. It breaks through mental blocks, dismantling the emotional block just as it dismantles encoded trauma blocks.

When you use Havening on mental blocks that sabotage your personal goals like procrastination, feeling unworthy or unmotivated, feeling unsuccessful or like a failure, it will automatically seek out and dismantle any encoded messages stored in the brain connected to these specific emotions, words or if there is a specific event that triggered these negative feelings.

When you use Havening on negative feelings you will be eradicating blocks and obstacles that sabotage your personal happiness.

Module 8: Strategies To Take Back Your Life

Pacing And Goal Setting

Pain usually leads to a change in activity levels. You may give up activities as a way to avoid pain. You may find that you push harder, determined, the pain will not stop you only to find that pushing harder can mean you get pain flareups from over-activity.

The pacing approach gives you a way to schedule rest periods and take a break every day. You can break activities into smaller bits to pace yourself, so you are doing little bits of activity often, and finding a common ground so that you are not overdoing it. Pacing helps you to stay more active and being able to do the things you care about. Pacing helps you pre-plan what you want and need to get done without overdoing it to cause a pain flareup.

Pacing Can Help You:

- Allows you to do more activities you enjoy
- Experience less pain flare ups from over activity
- Feel more in control of your pain levels

Pacing Has Two Benefits:

You can conserve energy for activities you value for example, playing with your kids, complete work projects or going to special events.
You can gradually start to increase activity levels to help you do more activities and to tolerate more so that eventually you become more active with less pain

Pacing is designed to be a tool you use to pre-plan activities, just like you plan for a vacation and plan what you will need to pack in a suitcase. Pacing should be used as a pain management strategy in combination with a doctor approved activity program to increase your activity levels.

Pacing uses a time contingent approach to activity rather than a pain contingent approach. This means an activity is based on measurement of the amount of time or the number of repetitions rather than how much pain it causes.

This type of measure gives you a target and a limit for the activity for example, 15 minutes of walking or 10 minutes of lighthouse work gives you a foundation from which to build up activity tolerance. This is important because it allows you to do more of your everyday activity without experiencing pain flare-ups.

How Do I Use Pacing

Prioritize the activities that you have to do today. Write them down, arrange in an order of priority, you can ask yourself if each task really needs to get done today and then cross off those that are not necessary. If there is one really important thing you need to do, arrange your pacing schedule around this task. Remember to make time for scheduled rest breaks.

Keep A Pain Diary Or Use A Pain App

You will find there is a wide variety of pain diary Apps used for Pacing. Find the App that best fits your lifestyle and needs. You will find the App does all the work for you in designing a pacing schedule. * NOTE: Please check with your doctor before changing exercise or activity levels.

Pacing Basics:

- Write down the time, distance, or number of times, that you can do the activity or task without a pain flare up.
- Set your baseline based on the most limiting symptoms and take three measures over three different days to give yourself the best guide.
- Take an average of these measures, add the three numbers together then divide by three you should then reduce this number by 20% just to give yourself a little buffer.
- You can calculate this number on your phone and keep track of it. They do have a wide variety of special pain apps to choose from that you may find useful and helping you to set your pacing goals.
- You can try to increase by 10% each week the amount of activity that you can do without pain flare ups, so you increase the time distance or the number of repetitions of each activity by 10%.

- You can set goals for yourself in pacing, working up to an activity that you want to be able to do take small amounts of activity do them often take breaks.
- You are going to take a regularly planned relaxation break when you pace even on the days when you feel good. It is essential to still rest so even though you are having a good day, you are still going to take your break.
- Plan short rest before and after a particularly stressful or demanding task.
- You practice relaxation stretching daily walks even on a not so good day because this helps you to control the pain.
- Some of the things you do not want to do in pacing: when pain gets in the way, it is a mistake to push through. Stop the activity.
- On a good day, do not do more than the pacing schedule allows.
- Have a plan and aim to change only one or two things at a time.
- Keep a record of what you are doing and how much you were doing; write it down in a pain diary.
- Alternate heavier task with lighter or less stressful ones.
- Use one kind of task as a break from another, change your body position and posture regularly.
- On a bad pain day, try to do some activities, but remember to be kind to yourself, rest when you need to rest.
- If you have had a flareup of pain, go back to a level that you can cope with activity and start pacing and building up again.

Pain Friendly Diet Suggestions

* NOTE: Be sure to check with your medical doctor before making any diet regimen changes

You are what you eat. The foods you eat play a major role in pain levels for most people with chronic pain syndromes. Researchers have found that an anti-inflammatory diet can help reduce inflammatory pain flareups. A low Histamine diet may also help, histamine creates inflammation in the body. Fresh foods and simple ingredients are best.

Keeping a food diary for 3 weeks may help you to determine what foods seem to trigger a painful reaction on that day or even into the next day. You may notice with certain foods that you have an increase in pain or you may be prone to insomnia. You would want to eliminate or reduce these foods.

The Food Diary

Keeping a food diary is simple. You will keep a notebook of what you eat through the course of the day including snacks and beverages. At the end of each day, you will take note of your pain levels and any additional symptoms like headaches, allergic type symptoms, GI digestive issues, depressed mood, insomnia or unusual fatigue.

Once you have several weeks of diary notes you will begin to see if there is a link between certain foods and any symptoms you may be experiencing. You can use the diary to show your doctor if there is any correlation.

Inflammatory foods you may want to avoid:

- Processed, fast foods chain restaurants, pre-cooked, packaged, canned foods
- Foods with "fake" sugar substitutes
- Unhealthy oils
- Processed carbs, which are present in white bread, white pasta, and many baked goods
- Processed snack foods, such as chips
- Premade high sugar desserts, cookies, candy, chocolate, soda
- Excess alcohol beverages

Gluten & Nightshade Vegetables: Some people may find it beneficial to limit their intake of the following foods: Dairy, Gluten along with nightshade vegetables. Plants belonging to the nightshade family, such as tomatoes, eggplants, peppers, and potatoes, seem to trigger flares in some people with inflammatory diseases. Carbohydrates: A high carb diet, even when the carbs are healthy, may promote inflammation in some people.

Low Histamine Diet: Histamine in foods can promote inflammation. Histamine exists in all foods. Following a low histamine diet can help reduce painful inflammatory flareups. You can find a variety of programs to suit your individual needs for a low histamine diet online.

Alkaline- normal pH level diet: Keeping the body at a normal alkaline pH level is important. A high acidic body can cause inflammation. You can find alkaline pH level diet books and charts online. Test your body every few days for pH level using test strips.

Foods That May Help Manage Inflammation:

- Oily fish, such as tuna and salmon
- Fruits, such as blackberries, blueberries, strawberries, and cherries
- Vegetables, including spinach, Kale, and broccoli
- Nuts and seeds
- Olives and olive oil
- Fiber
- Raw or moderately cooked vegetables
- Legumes, such as lentils
- Spices, such as turmeric and ginger
- Probiotics and prebiotics
- Green tea

Exercise: List the diet changes you will need to make to lower inflammation.

Know Your Pain Triggers

Can you name your three top pain triggers? Mine are stress, over activity and the damp weather. Using a pain diary can help you discover what causes a flare-up in your symptoms. Keeping a pain diary may help you make discoveries of triggers you may be are unaware of.

You will find a variety of Pain Diary Apps available. Some are disease specific written especially for CRPS or Fibromyalgia. Knowing what triggers, a pain flare-up is an important part of managing pain. Some of these triggers, we can do nothing about like the weather, but others like stress and over-activity we can manage. We can use Pacing Activity Programs to pre-plan activities and find effective stress management programs to help control stress.

Stress and emotional upset can cause flare-ups in most chronic pain syndromes. When we are stressed, our muscles are tight and tense, causing even more pain. Stress triggers the "fight or flight response" in the body releasing hormones that can create inflammation in the body.

Stress is a part of life, but we can counter its effects by using natural drug-free relaxation therapies:

- Retrain Your Brain therapy techniques
- Guided imagery for stress control
- Progressive muscle relaxation (use the Inner Sanctuary script)
- Mindfulness meditation practices
- Yoga, tai-chi, qi-gong exercise
- Walking in nature, light exercise,
- Crafts and hobbies to distract the mind
- Cognitive Behavioral "talk" Therapy
- Selfcare programs that nourish the mind, body, and soul

Practice Exercise:

1. List your pain triggers (stress, activity, environment or places, people, foods, weather)
2. When are they most likely to be triggered
3. Review your list; is there a common denominator or theme to your pain triggers
4. What mind-body tool will you use to reduce or eliminate your pain triggers

Healthy Sleep

Getting deep restorative peaceful sleep is important for people with chronic pain and illness. Pain-insomnia is a real condition that most people in chronic pain experience at one time or another. Deep REM sleep is a vital component to healing our bodies. Try natural relaxation methods like listening to the Recordable Meditation Therapy Script at bedtime for deep relaxation. If you feel the insomnia is pain-induced, try the NLP pain relief techniques before bedtime.

Improving your sleep may require retraining your brain to fall asleep and stay asleep longer for sound restorative sleep

The Swish Technique found in this book can be used for insomnia to release the old behavior pattern of insomnia and pave a new neural pathway for sound restorative sleep. Practice the Swish Technique for insomnia, stress, anxiety or fears.

Good sleep behaviors may also play a role in peaceful sleep.

- Create the right conditions in a peaceful relaxed place that induces sleep.
- Control the lighting, most people sleep better in a dark room, filter noise so the room is quiet with no disruptions, a cool room temperature and a comfortable mattress may be key to solving insomnia. Some people sleep better with white noise; sounds of white noise, nature or ocean sounds while sleeping.
- Develop a regular sleep routine: same time to bed, same time waking in the morning. Start a regular bedtime routine: where you give your mind and body time to wind-down from the day's stress or activities. Perhaps a relaxing bath before bed to relax the muscles and quiet the mind. Eliminate watching TV in the bedroom.

- Avoid caffeine, alcohol and cigarettes several hours before bedtime. If you go to bed after eating a big meal, digestive issues like acid reflux may be what keeps you awake.
- Manage stress so a worried mind does not keep you awake. If you are feeling troubled and cannot quiet your mind to sleep, try writing it all down, start journaling to get the emotions out, keeping a gratitude journal by writing down the things you are grateful for in your life has been proven to help reduce anxiety and worry.
- Practice mindfulness meditation.

If you have tried natural methods and are still having trouble sleeping talk to your doctor for recommendations.

Practice Exercise: Set up your own healthy sleep plan

1. What changes will you make to create a peaceful sleep environment?
2. What new sleep routine will you incorporate?
3. How will you soothe and relax the mind-body before bedtime?

Self-Care

Selfcare is a form of healthcare. It is not a luxury, and it is not being egotistical of selfish to take loving care of yourself. When you have chronic pain and illness, taking loving care of yourself must be your top priority. Developing a regular organized plan of Selfcare is essential to your overall health and well-being. In general, the goals of self-care are to find a state of good mental and physical health, reduce stress, meet emotional needs and find a balance in one's life.

The benefits of Self-care are numerous. A regular program gives you emotional resiliency and can help you cope with stress better. Self-care activities are self-empowering, it restores and replenishes during and after stressful periods. It can help you to better cope with the challenges that living with chronic pain and illness presents on a daily basis. Self-care brings out the best in ourselves. It is an act of self-love, a form of compassionate healing for our own self. It has been medically proven that when people participate in their own care program, it builds self-confidence in their ability to manage their health conditions better. It puts you back in charge.

I define Self-care as any intentional action that you take to nourish the soul and take care of your physical, mental, emotional and spiritual health. A Self-care program should be designed to fit your own personal needs. There are not any one-size fits all approach to developing a plan of care.

Self-care is as individual as we are. For people with chronic pain and illness the plan is as individual as the pain and illness we experience. What is pain-relieving and soothing to one person may not be for another. Self-care can be especially challenging for people with chronic pain, illness and disabilities. You may need to seek assistance to complete an organized plan.

Some people find it overwhelming to take on too many new things all at once, start gradually with a couple of your top priorities to get the important care that you need and build on that. Health professionals often use the term self-care to refer to one's ability to take care of the activities of daily living, or ADLs, such as feeding oneself, showering, brushing one's teeth, wearing clean clothes, and attending to medical concerns but Self-care is actually much more than just ADL, it is nourishing the mind body and soul.

3 Key Selfcare Components To Whole Person Wellness

Modern selfcare nourishes the whole person, addressing your mental, physical, emotional and spiritual needs. It is simply taking the time to give yourself what you need. We all have different requirements for self-care and that is why it is so important to create your own personalized plan of care.

You will find that the plan may need to be adjusted and changed over time to accommodate life changes. You may focus your activities on ADL or basic activities of daily living while at other times you need to nourish the soul and feel pampered. Sometimes it will be about what you need right now in the moment.

Create Your Own Self-Care Plan

Start creating your own personalized Self-care plan by incorporating the things you love to do. CAM Complimentary-Alternative therapies, walks on the beach, reading a book and doing your favorite hobby or craft can be a form of nourishing self-care. Anything that allows you to mentally escape mental stress is a good selfcare activity. It does not need to cost money, it can be a simple walk-in nature or watching your favorite movie comedy that makes you laugh.

Plan Self-care activities on a regular basis. You may find setting up a monthly plan by setting aside specific time in advance for activities works best.

Exercise: Create a Selfcare plan for the week

Start your plan by asking yourself a couple of simple questions. You may want to start a self-care notebook and write your answers down on paper. These answers may change over time. Review your plan every three-six month or as you need to update it.

- What do I need most right now? Physically, mentally, emotionally and spiritually?
- What do I want?
- What will make me feel better right now?

If you feel setting up your own Self-care program is overwhelming, you can find a variety of books and Apps available to help get you started on a regular plan of care.

Pain Support Groups

A chronic pain support group provides a forum for people to be able to talk about their pain and not feel so isolated or alone in their pain. It is common for people in chronic pain to feel isolated or alienated from families, not able to talk about their pain, and frustrated by the lack of medical care or services.

There is usually a sense of community and compassion to support meetings and it is also a time for learning and sharing. You may learn about different therapies or techniques or strategies that will be able to help you to manage your pain better.

You may be able to find disease specific groups for people with Fibromyalgia, Lyme Disease, CRPS, Gout that have the same condition as you.

You will find camaraderie among people; friendships usually develop because you have so much in common with the other people in the group. They get it- they understand what it is to live in pain. They know the rollercoaster ride of emotions that you go through day-to-day.

The American Chronic Pain Association has support groups in all 50 states their focus is not on symptoms or applying treatments but on helping you manage pain better, supporting you. You should find a group you are comfortable in, one that really offers compassion and understanding and is uplifting for you. There are many different ones and so if you go to one and you do not feel that it is the right fit for you find another one that does.

You can find many support groups online that offer Zoom-type meetings. I actually think that is more convenient for pain people to attend a support group in the comfort of their own home.

Module 9: Recordable Meditation Therapy Scripts

Recordable Meditation Therapy Scripts are a breakthrough treatment in selfcare regimens. They are more effective than listening to pre-recorded audios MP3's and they empower people by taking an active role in their own wellness program. Listening to the therapy script nightly reinforces the positive changes you desire as it creates new neuropathways for positive change.

Recordable Scripts Vs Mp3 Audio Downloads

Using your own voice in recorded scripts is the key to highly effective therapy. Neurosciences has proven that listening to your own voice is more effective than listening to a pre-recorded MP3 download using a stranger's voice. Your subconscious mind knows your own voice. It recognizes and responds to your voice immediately, without hesitation, it accepts the symbols and suggestions as truth, as real because it is being instructed to do so by your own voice. It acts on the mind-body instructions without question. Your voice is extremely powerful whether it is used for positive affirmations or on a recorded therapy audio. It results in quicker, more successful therapy outcomes.

How To Record The Therapy Scripts

7 Easy Steps:
1) First: read the recordable therapy script out loud before recording it so you get comfortable with the wording and pauses (practice it before recording so you read it smoothly).
2) Set up your recording device (if using your phone turn the ringer to quiet).
3) Make sure the recording room is quiet with no outside noises so you will not be disturbed while recording.
4) Do a test for voice is at the right volume setting.

5) If you want relaxing music in the background, choose a soothing instrumental that has the right pacing to your speech. (You can purchase background music with just instrumentals to download online).
6) Read the script into the recording device, slowly, with a soothing voice.
7) When finished, save it, give it a title. (you may want to make a second copy in case the first gets deleted accidentally).

Recording Tips

Read through the script completely before recording it. When recording the scripts, you want to use a calm, soft, relaxing voice. Talk slowly, use pauses to give yourself time to do the imagery and visualizations. Do not be afraid to make a mistake-read through and practice the script before you record it. I have capitalized some words you may want to emphasize while speaking. I use (...) to indicate a pause in the sentencing.

TIP: I like to use soothing instrumental background music on my recordings. I find it more relaxing.

Do Not Change The Wording Or Phrases In The Scripts. You May Change The Therapeutic Outcome

Do not add or change the wording, symbols, or imagery in the script. Do not shorten the length of the script. You may be changing the therapeutic outcomes. NLP Practitioners are trained in linguistics (wording), creating correct verbal suggestions or symbols that trigger the subconscious mind to take action by incorporating the correct symbols that the subconscious mind will accept and act upon. The script is written by a professional and will have the appropriate NLP suggestions and techniques to help you achieve your goals.

How To Use The Recordings For The Most Benefit

The scripts are meant to be read into a voice recorder like the one on your mobile phone or tablet so that you can have the convenience of using the recordings whenever and wherever you want.

The recordings are meant to be used in a relaxed, quiet setting where you can relax and daydream using the therapeutic images, symbols, and visualizations. Use headphones to mentally tune-in and avoid distraction.

The best time to listen to the recording is at bedtime, where you simply drift off into peaceful sleep while listening to the recording. Do not worry if you fall asleep during the recording, it is more beneficial, remember your subconscious mind is most dominant during sleep and will absorb and act upon the suggestions more readily.

Important Warning: Do not listen to the recordings while driving the car or doing any activity that requires your alert attention.

The recordings can make you drowsy they may distract you causing accidents. NLP, hypnosis, guided imagery, mediations, visualizations are designed to be relaxing and can distract your attention. They can make you drowsy or sleepy. They have the most benefit when used in a quiet relaxed setting.

Module 10: Therapy Script #1 - For CRPS

Recordable Script For CRPS
(Pain Relief written specifically for CRPS-Complex Regional Pain Syndrome
Recordable script for CRPS by Carol Charland
*All Copyrights Reserved 2023

Follow the instructions for recording the scripts.

START RECORDING HERE (Read Slowly – With A Soothing Voice)

Please DO NOT Listen to this recording while driving the car of doing any activity that requires your alert attention.

Get into a quiet place so you can relax without being interrupted.

Begin by taking in three deep cleansing breaths and exhale all the way out into your abdomen.
Simply relaxing and letting go with each breath that you take... let your body sink down into a relaxing comfort.

I want you to use your imagination and daydream, just as if you were on a wonderful vacation.

Picture yourself on a warm, sunny beach it can be any beach that you would like... perhaps it's a warm tropical place that you've always dreamed of traveling to... or a favorite beach that you've been to before- use all your senses to place yourself in this daydream. Imagine the sights, sounds, smells...

This will be known as your "favorite place" it's your own *Inner Sanctuary* where you can escape to relax, let go of stress, tension, pain or discomfort.

Picture all the sights and sounds of this beautiful beach. Use all your senses to actually place yourself there -you can imagine yourself walking down the beach... feeling the soft sand on your feet... not a care in the world, stress-free, carefree and relaxed. With each breath you relax deeper and deeper... just letting your mind wander into the daydream.

You can smell the fresh salt air... feel the warmth of the sun on your face... and there's a gentle breeze blowing through your hair... you see the crystal clear water with sparkling beams of sunlight dancing across the waves... it looks so refreshing... and you hear the rhythmic sounds of the waves as they roll into shore, in and out... the golden beams of sunlight on your face is so relaxing... you let yourself sink down deeper into the relaxation... all your muscles letting go... relaxing... it feels so good to relax... let go... escape for a little while...

Close your eyes... and feel the warm golden beams of sunlight on your face and body... sparkling beams of solar radiance... you breathe them in... and send them thru your mind and body... relaxing with each breath... breathing normally... easily... in and out...

I want you to imagine small, sparkling balls of golden energy... like beams of sunlight... you breath them in send them throughout your body... and as you exhale your breath... you are going to move the sparkling balls of energy...little beams of sunlight... thru your body... imagine that they clear a path... like a snowplow- plowing snow... clears away fatigue, tiredness, clearing away any old energy... old mental and physical stress, tension, clearing away any discomfort mentally, physically or emotionally... from the mind and body... clearing a path for new fresh energy... vitality... clearing and restoring all the energy pathways, meridians, to new... fresh life force energy and vitality.

Imagine the golden ball of energy like beams of sunlight are sitting at the very top of your head... With your breath as you exhale... you can move this warm flow of energy... golden beams of sunlight flow down over your forehead... relaxing all the muscles across your forehead... over your eyelids... and around your eyes... relax all the muscles in your face, it flows down into your jaw... and all the muscles in your jaw relax... flows down your throat ... and it seems to flow right down into your shoulders... relaxing... flowing down your arms... clearing a path for fresh new energy... down into your wrist... and down into your hands and fingers... just imagine you can the warm flow of sunshine ... flow right out through your fingertips... you are letting go of stress and tension... any pain and discomfort leaving your body... its clearing a path...

You can feel that flow of warm golden beams of sunlight flowing down your chest... it surrounds your heart... it feels so soothing and comforting, loving... and it flows into your abdomen... softening the muscles... so warm and comforting... relaxing all the muscles in your abdomen...

As it flows down into your hips... down into your thighs... and legs... clearing a path... into your feet and toes... now, imagine that on the very ends of your toes there are these magical drains... and you are letting this warm flow of golden beams of sunlight flow right out through the very ends of your toes... out through the drains... all the stress, tension, any pain or discomfort is leaving your body... as you relax more and more. Letting go...

You can imagine yourself letting go of any stress or tension right out through those magical drains anytime that you need to... let your body deeply relax now... sinking down into the comfort of your own body.

Now... imagine those golden beams of sunlight filling your spinal column... like a golden tube of sparkling light... from the tailbone... the base of your spine... it flows upward... filling your spine... with healing energy... healing all the nerves in the spinal column... it flows upward... between the shoulder blades...up into the back of your neck... and the base of your skull... warm soothing, healing golden beams of sparkling light... you can feel that warmth relaxing all of the muscles in your back... in your neck... healing all the nerves in the spine... healing the Vagus nerve, the Central Nervous system... the Autonomic Nervous System... the Sympathetic and Para-sympathetic system...   take a moment and see the spinal column... a golden tube of healing light... healing all the nerves... relax and absorb this healing light...

Imagine the warm flow of sunlight moves up the back of your head... to the very top of your head... where it stays for a moment...   the golden light surrounds your head... it is absorbed by your brain, your mental functions and emotions... its healing your emotional body... restoring mental function, clarity, focus, memory... you easily let go of any mental stress, mental tension...calming and soothing the brain... the warm soothing light simply absorbs it all... you feel clear-headed, brain-fog is gone... you easily focus... have mental clarity to make wise choices and decisions... all mental function is restored to normal...

Once again you can let that warm flow of sunlight flow down over your face... and it feels so warm and soothing and relaxing...all the muscles in your jaw relaxing... It flows down into your chest and abdomen... just imagine that this golden sparkling light comes to rest in your abdomen... right above your navel... this is its home...

Just imagine you can throw out an anchor... grounding your energy... you feel safe, secure, grounded... centered and in complete balance... this is feeling of a deep inner strength... you can tap into it whenever you need to... you feel grounded, centered, balanced, secure and stable.

You've just made this complete circle from the top of your head to the tips of your toes... with little golden beams of solar radiance... restoring vital life force... healing energy to the mind and body... you've brought this life force energy back to rest... in the abdomen... where it gives you deep inner strength...

You have just completed a technique for natural relaxation called *Progressive Relaxation* where you relax all the muscles from the top of your head to tips of your toes... when you relax muscles, any tight tense muscles from pain are released... you practice this technique to relax the muscles... progressive relaxation helps you release pain.

In Chinese-Taoist medicine this technique is known as the *"Circle Of Life"* moving life force energy to clear away old stale energy, any blocks to wellness, you are restoring the flow of natural vital, life-force energy that restores and heals the body... it automatically brings a renewed sense of health and well-being, fresh energy, strength and vitality. It strengthens your mind and body.

You can practice this breathing technique anytime that you would like... releasing stress, tension, pain or discomfort from the mind and body. You will always feel a deep inner strength... restored mind and body... energized

---

(The release technique)

Return to the daydream now... walking down the beach I want you to imagine that you can see the most perfect place to sit down and relax for a moment... I want you to picture in your mind a hammock... you're going to sit down and relax a while in the hammock... you can feel the gentle swaying motion of the hammock... it's so relaxing and soothing... as you swing back and forth... back and forth you feel the warmth of sunlight on your face... and you breathe and relax... stress-free... you notice the blueness of the sky above... there's some white soft fluffy clouds scattered across the sky... you relax deeper and deeper...

While you're relaxing in the hammock... we're going to begin to make a little **mental checklist** about CRPS ... any painful symptoms that you may be experiencing in regard to the CRPS...
 this is just as if you are writing it all down on a list in your mind... it's a mental checklist

First- I want you to go back into your memory, I want you to put down on this list when you **first experienced the symptoms** of the CRPS... was it after an injury, fall, surgery, trauma, whatever it is that "you think" is **the root cause** of the CRPS... whether it is known or unknown to you. (your subconscious mind knows the root cause and will put it on the list for you)

So put everything on the list about your injury and the onset of CRPS... when... where...

Next- I want you to put down on this list the **symptoms** that you have been experiencing in regard to the area effected by CRPS...   pain, swelling, discoloration of the skin, bruising, sweating, the sensitivity to touch or discomfort of blankets, clothing or shoes touching the skin... temperature changes- hot or cold- maybe it's both. Any inflammation, bone pain, muscle tightness or cramping, weakness... the inability to use the affected limb- lack of mobility or function, distorted shape... now add any other symptom you think needs to be there.

And... put down some of the **other additional symptoms** you may experience- like hyper-sensitivity to loud noises, bright lights, smells, or ringing in the ears. The inability to get deep sleep- insomnia. Any anxiety... PTSD symptoms, Hyper-vigilance or the busy mind that doesn't shut off. A sensory overload in the brain... fatigue and tiredness, any digestive or bowel problems, headaches, brain fog or memory problems, allergies, low immune system function. Add any <u>symptoms</u> to the list.

We know that CRPS is a <u>malfunction of the sympathetic nervous system</u> that can also involve the <u>malfunction of the Autonomic and Central Nervous System</u>- so put these malfunctions of the nervous systems on the list.

Add… any **emotional symptoms** like stress, tension, feeling overwhelmed, depression, grief or sadness at being in pain and disabled, loss of your old lifestyle, anger, anxiety, emotional exhaustion…

Add any emotional symptom – if you cannot put a name to a feeling you are having- just put a square box on the list… to represent this unknown feeling… -now add whatever you feel needs to be on the list.

Describe the CRPS pain "sensation" … and discomfort- is it <u>burning</u> neuropathy, is it <u>sharp</u>, dull, achy, deep bone pain, muscle tightness or cramping… add whatever you like.

List what causes additional pain- any pain or discomfort with weather changes… pain with activity… with movement or use of the limb… standing… walking… weather. add whatever you like

Some medical experts think that CRPS is caused by old, out-dated pain messages sent to the brain and for some reason they got "stuck" there… like an old out-dated <u>cassette tape player</u> that broke, and the tape is stuck repeating the same message.

We're going to use pictures and symbols in this release technique to work with the part of the brain that stores these old-outdated… CRPS pain messages… we're instructing the brain to release them… it is easy to do… to just let them go… your subconscious already knows how to do this…

You realize you don't need or want these old messages about pain or discomfort any longer. You're ready to let them go and be free of pain or discomfort...

I want you to <u>picture an old tape player</u>... and you can see that its broken... the tape is stuck in it. This is what "YOUR" <u>CRPS pain messaging</u> looks like... you can see the messages stuck on the tape. Put a label on the tape messages... "pain messages" Now, I want you to imagine taking the stuck tape of messages- out of the tape recorder... its actually is quite easy to do... just rip it out,
THEN you can throw the old broken tape recorder away- it's no good any longer.

Now- I want you to imagine you can <u>put that tape of pain messages</u>... on the <u>mental checklist</u> that you are making about CRPS. Do it now. <u>Picture the image of the tape on the list.</u>

Now- you have everything you need on this mental checklist about CRPS... (don't worry your subconscious mind knows what needs to be there to help you achieve your goal of being pain free and free of CRPS)

Put the mental checklist aside for just a moment... and return to the daydream of the warm sunny beach... walking down the beach, relaxing. Breathe and relax... Taking in all the sights and sounds of your favorite place. Simply breath and relax for a moment....

At the end of the beach, you notice a <u>beautiful, hot-air balloon with a basket attached</u>- (you can make it be any color you would like) – the hot air balloon and basket is tied down to the beach with 3 silver cords.

Picture yourself standing in front of the basket of the hot-air balloon.

I want you to use your imagination… gather up the <u>mental checklist you just made about CRPS</u>.

That's right- picture yourself putting everything on the list into the basket.

- All the reasons why you might have ever gotten CRPS, the trauma, injury or root cause of why you got CRPS- known or unknown to you…
- All the pain, symptoms… additional symptoms and any emotional symptoms… any pain causing activity,
- The description of CRPS pain… burning, sharp…
- Toss in the nervous systems malfunctioning… and any health problems it might have caused…
- And finally, Toss in the tape from the old tape recorder. the pain messaging tape… with those messages on it.
- Picture yourself tossing the tape into the basket- now.
- Ask your subconscious mind to add anything to the basket that needs to be there…

You're going to put all this stuff… anything that has to do with CRPS or pain and discomfort into the basket of the hot-air balloon… do it now.

<u>Everything… is in the basket that needs to be there about crps</u> … don't worry if you think you might have forgotten something… your subconscious mind knows what needs to be there and will include it to help you achieve your goal…

So, you can take a moment and breathe and relax… in and out… easily…

NOW- I want you to imagine… in your hand… you have a pair of golden scissors…

You are going to cut the 3 silver cords… that holds the basket and hot-air balloon to the ground on the count of 3.

Do that now. Cut the cords. Count #1… cut the cord. #2… cut the cord. #3… cut the cord.
All right- you did it… Good job, you can relax now.

NOW- breathe and relax as you watch the hot-air balloon and basket float up into the blue sky.
…quickly and effortlessly up into the blue sky… there are some white soft fluffy clouds… a warm breeze is carrying it away… up higher than the clouds… and before you know it… it fades from your view… and its GONE. GONE permanently - never to return.

Completely gone… faded from your view. The hot-air balloon and basket has been carried away on that warm breeze… never to return. So… you can relax now… your work is done.

Take in a deep cleansing breath and exhale all the way out… like a big sigh of relief.

You have set yourself free… from the CRPS and pain messages, and any of the symptoms of it… and anything that has to do with CRPS…

Your subconscious mind is going to use this simple release technique … to release and let go of any of the trauma, pain or symptoms… from past or present… it has released any of the root causes of why you might have ever experienced CRPS and chronic pain… it has released the symptoms… and it does it immediately, easily and without hesitation…

Trust that your subconscious mind knows what to do with the symbols, pictures and suggestions to help you achieve your goal of releasing CRPS… chronic pain and symptoms… completely.

You don't even have to think about it… the subconscious knows what to do with the pictures and suggestions and releases it ALL… automatically.

Now take a moment to breathe… imagine yourself basking in the warm sunlight on the beach.

You have set yourself FREE… that's right FREE… from pain or discomfort… free from CRPS and any of its symptoms. It's simply gone.

You can imagine yourself "jumping for joy" that's right go ahead… be happy… feel the freedom…feel the rush of excitement fill your mind and body… you have set yourself FREE.

You can now bask in that feeling of complete freedom… it feels wonderful…

Once again, return to the daydream… Imagine yourself walking down the beach… happier than ever before… joyful… you feel lighter… free, wonderful, happy… healthy… you are free of crps pain and discomfort… its simply gone.

Your body will begin to immediately adjust to this new reality… free from CRPS… free from pain or discomfort… the pain fades away to nothing… the swelling disappears… the bruising and discoloration fades away… the CRPS limb/body parts return to normal movement and function.

You return to a normal, healthy state... as if you have always been healthy. Remember Dr Herbert Benson's *Remembered Wellness technique* Your subconscious mind holds the blueprint of your perfect health... you can return to perfect health... imagine that now.

Repeat These Affirmations-
- I now act-feel and think- FREE OF CRPS PAIN- as if I have always been- free of pain.
- I have set myself free... I have the power to set myself free from pain and discomfort...
- Each and every day, I feel better and better in every way... healthier and happier
- My mind and body return to a high level of health and wellness... naturally
- I now experience complete remission of the CRPS, and any co-conditions associated with it.
- I know that my mind-body knows how to do this... I don't even have to think about it. It does it all on its own... effortlessly, immediately... and without hesitation.
- I am self-confident in my healing...

(PAUSE FOR A MOMENT)

We will now be using powerful techniques to instruct the mind-body using the Role Modeling Technique.

Relax... breathe... use your imagination... Picture the original health blueprint for your body free of pain, injury or illness.

Now- I want you to go back in your memory and picture yourself before the CRPS... before injury, pain or symptoms, before illness or disease.

Take a moment to get a clear picture... you can almost feel it... when you were healthy and well

You can remember what it is like to be healthy and well.

See the perfect image of yourself... from the master blueprint... age does not matter... it's the image and feeling you have of being healthy... that you remember... you know how to be healthy and well... and how to act-feel- and think pain-free and healthy... as if you have always been.

So, get a good image of yourself in your mind and the feel of yourself healthy. You may even have a photograph of yourself healthy... so you can picture this image of yourself

<u>Now</u> use your imagination... you are on the beach... go back to your favorite place *The Inner Sanctuary*... feeling the warm sunshine, relaxing, daydreaming... walking down the beach...

<u>And</u>... right in front of you is the perfect image of you... in a healthy body- free of pain, illness or discomfort...

<u>Next</u>... I want you to imagine you can simply step-into the image in front of you...step into your healthy body... before pain or illness... imagine being free of CRPS, free of pain or discomfort...

Imagine your body just melting and merging into this healthy image... from the top of your head down to the tips of your toes... down your arms to your hands and fingers... you melt and merge into the healthy body... your subconscious mind knows how to do this... it feels so real to you... because you are engaging your memory... it remembers this level of wellness... it knows how to do this... and it wants to do this... your mind-body wants to heal itself... and now you have given it the tool to do so...

Take a moment, breathe and relax... so, you can feel this level of health, wellness, energy returning to your body... feel it in every part of your body, every cell, fiber, nerve, muscle... you remember... you know this feeling... its wonderful... you can really feel it... with each breath this sense of wellness gets stronger and stronger... you feel healthier and healthier in every way.

Just breathe... relax and sink down into the comfort of your body... It feels wonderful... you remember... you know what wellness is... relax and breathe... bask in the feeling... know its permanent.

Imagine flipping an inner switch... flip it to free of pain. Lock it in place.

You now hold <u>the key</u> to the self-healing mechanism in your mind-body. You have unlocked the healing potential that we all possess...

You are in complete control... You take control of your own healing... your health and wellness...

Picture yourself holding a large golden key... you successfully have unlocked the healing potential of your mind-body... you are in complete control. You feel self-confident, empowered and you sense a deep inner strength... coming to the surface... it feels wonderful... you are taking back your life from the grip of pain, illness or discomfort... You feel healthier than you ever have...

See yourself exactly the way you want to be... imagine that you have returned to a state of perfect health... the blueprint... (before you ever had crps or any illness)

You will now act- feel- and think- in perfect health, free of crps pain, free of discomfort or illness... as if you have always been free of CRPS... you enjoy perfect health.

You are in complete control… you hold the key… you intuitively know what you need to do… to return to perfect health… to the blueprint… and you do it… And so, it is… healed and healthy… healed and healthy

And… breathe and relax… your work is done now…

(you will use this easy role modeling technique of "Remembered Wellness" each day- you take a few moments to get quiet, relax… and picture your mind-body healthy and well.)

The Dashboard: We will now use the powerful symbol of the NLP dashboard- so picture in your mind a dashboard or control center and imagine this is the control center for your mind-body.

We truly do have a control center in our mind… and it is said… if you speak to the mind… the body will follow- we just need to give it instructions.

We are going to use the symbols of dials and switches on your mind-body dashboard to instruct the body.

On the dashboard you can picture different gauges, dials, switches and knobs…

The Pain Dial … you see a **bright orange-red like a flame dial** on the master control panel of your mind and body… it has a label on it that says…. **PAIN.**

The dial has numbers from 10 to zero (the same as the pain scale has) So the dial is set at 10… start to turn the dial down… you may even want to count to yourself as we turn it down to 9—let the pain fade away… 8—7—6—5—count down lower and lower turn it down fading the pain to nothing… 4—3—2—1- and finally to 0—zero.

Zero being no pain at all- (just like on the pain scale) you have successfully turned down pain- or any discomfort to ZERO... ZERO on the pain scale. Now lock it in place at zero. You are free of CRPS pain and discomfort. The pain scale is at ZERO.

Next, you will see a power switch that has the label **Insomnia** (restless sleep) ... I want you to turn that switch **OFF.** Just like turning OFF a light switch... when you turn your bedroom lights OFF... you are programming your mind-body for sleep. Telling it that at your given bedtime- it is time to sleep Picture that in your mind now- when you turn OFF your bedroom light at bedtime you are instructing your body for sound peaceful healing sleep.

Affirmations For Peaceful Sound Sleep

- I fall to sleep easily at my given bedtime, I stay asleep throughout the night.
- If I should need to awaken during the night, I will do so... and handle anything I need to... And I will be able to return to sound peaceful sleep when I return to bed.
- I awaken in the morning feeling refreshed, well rested, and ready to start my day.
- I now enjoy sound peaceful sleep... I sleep like a baby... peacefully throughout the night.
- I fall to sleep easily at my given bedtime and remain a sleep until it is time to wake in the morning, at my given time.
- I get deep sound peaceful sleep that heals my body, restores my health... and replenishes my energy.
- When I awaken in the morning, I feel well rested, energized and ready to start my day... I am free from CRPS... chronic pain or illness... today and everyday... from this day forward.

- Each and every day, I notice how much better I feel... better and better in every way... healthier, happier and completely well.

Next on the dashboard...   There is a **green gauge** that is labeled **HEALTH**... turn it to the high setting- <u>healed and healthy</u>. You have a high level of health and well-being.

Repeat to yourself- I am healed and healthy, healed and healthy, I am healed and healthy.

You will notice that any of the old symptoms of CRPS have been released... you are completely free of pain, symptoms... free of any discomfort or disease... you have now returned to a high level of health and well-being. Healed and Healthy.

Remission: see a power switch with the label on it that says **REMISSION.** Turn that power switch ON- full power. You are in complete remission...there are no visible signs of CRPS... you are pain-free... symptom-free... in full and complete remission. today and everyday...

See the **red gauge**...turn it to the setting **Crps Symptom Free**... you act- feel and think as if you have always been healed and healthy. Free of any of the CRPS symptoms, healed and healthy.

The next item on the dashboard is a giant **golden knob labeled STRESS**... that has numbers from 10- to-1.

Turn that knob down to a setting that feels right to you... just where it needs to be... where you are in complete control of stress... so that you can easily cope and manage with life's ups and downs. Stress bounces right off you like a bouncing rubber ball. It does not matter what happens in life... you make wise decisions... you think clearly, can focus, feel grounded, balanced and centered… you can handle any stress or situation that comes your way in a calm relaxed manner.

Stress-free, relaxed and calm. Breathe in the relaxation, feel the strength… you find healthy ways to cope and manage with stress… better than you ever have before.

Next on the dashboard- picture a **dark blue dial** that has a label "**fight or flight" anxiety**… and I want you to turn that to the setting that says **NORMAL**   Your sympathetic and para-sympathetic nervous system is in complete balance and harmony… it is normal.

You are naturally calmer and more relaxed now. You experience less anxiety. You find you have healthy coping mechanisms… You easily find healthy ways to relax …naturally.

If you should feel any signs of anxiety… you simply take in 3 deep cleansing breaths and relax… with each exhale... like a big sigh… releasing any stress or tension… clearing your mind and body of stress with the exhales… your mind and body relax…

You drink plenty of fresh water… you will find that water is a natural relaxant for you… when you drink water you feel calmer and more relaxed…   stress-free, any anxiety is washed away naturally.

See the **orange knob** that is labeled **emotionally strong and resilient**… turn that knob all the way up to the setting that says **DEEP INNER STRENGTH**. You are emotionally strong and resilient. You have deep inner strength that carries you through any situation… it does not matter what stress may come your way… you experience deep inner strength to cope and manage with life's ups and downs… you are emotionally strong… and resilient.

You can now easily cope and manage with anything that comes your way... in a clam relaxed manner... Always... Emotionally strong and resilient.

*Now... Lock it in place. Emotionally strong... deep inner strength.

Picture a light **blue switch** with the label... **BRAIN FOG** turn that switch **OFF**. You now are free of any mental or emotional confusion... forgetfulness or brain fog. You enjoy mental clarity, focus and concentration.

Next imagine a **silver gauge** labeled **IMMUNE SYSTEM** – turn the immune system up... give it a healthy boost..._turn it up a higher.... To a **STRONG** setting... where you know you have a strong healthy immune system that helps fight off disease, it helps stabilize your health and function of your body.

You'll notice a **cool blue lever**... labeled **ENDORPHINS**... endorphins are a brain chemical that is your body's natural pain reliever- said to be stronger than morphine or an opiate ... turn this lever to the **AUTOMATIC** position that reads **NATURAL PAIN RELIEF** Put it at the perfect place... just where it needs to be for pain relief- automatically.

See a yellow switch with the label **BODY FUNCTIONS**... flip that switch to NORMAL. All your organs, organ systems, nervous systems and body functions are now in complete balance and harmony and support your high level of health and wellness.

Along with the body function switch... there is a switch that reads the **NERVOUS SYSTEM**... the nervous system is like the electrical wiring in house... that keeps everything functioning properly... so, I want you to see a switch.... you will turn to NORMAL

Perfect balance and harmony... so that your nervous system; the central nervous system... the autonomic system... the Vagus nerve... the sympathetic and para-sympathetic nervous system... are all functioning normally and in perfect balance and harmony... to bring you perfect health.

Next there are **3 RED switches in a row**... labeled **DEPRESSION... SADNESS & GRIEF ... and ANGER**

Turn all 3 switches **OFF**... just like turning off a light switch... turn the power **OFF**.

Turn off **DEPRESSION**. Turn off sadness and grief. Turn off Anger and any negative emotion.

These negative emotions no longer have any power over you. Lock it in place-- OFF.

There is one final switch you will turn **ON**— it says **JOY AND HAPPINESS**... the switch is beautiful **pink rose colored switch**... it's time to turn that switch **ON.** Go ahead it's time for you to bring joy and happiness back into your life.

Imagine it's like turning ON the lights in a room where everything is brightly illuminated... it has a beautiful pink glow to it. Lock it in place.

Take a moment... surround yourself with love, joy, happiness... like wrapping yourself in a beautiful rose-colored bubble... Picture the new life you will have with more love, joy and happiness in it...
what is your heart's desire...? now that you have set yourself FREE...

You Realize... You have every switch, dial, gauge and knob on the mind-body control center-exactly where they need to be... to bring to you perfect health-- mentally, physically, emotionally...

Picture the control center- it's set perfectly.

The next imagery we will use to communicate to the mind-body uses **NLP sub-modalities** and it uses symbols and metaphors to communicate to the subconscious mind.

The First technique allows you to play with a symbol in order to change it...

I want you to <u>describe </u>CRPS pain as a burning sensation... so give it a symbol like a fire or flame. It is contained in a box...

You might even want to label the box CRPS pain or discomfort...

Now... what would you use to put out a fire or flame... a fire extinguisher? Or perhaps it is more like a big fire truck with a big fire hose of gushing water to put out the flame...
use a symbol (one that your mind sends you) to put the CRPS flame out... that's right... you are going to put the flame OUT. Do it now. Use the fire hose or extinguisher...
Imagine the flame is getting smaller... smaller.... fading... fading away to nothing... until the flame is completely out... it's been put out... extinguished completely.

You can throw the CRPS box out now. It's gone... completely gone. Great job.

NLP Anchor Technique- We will begin to use the symbol of water for an NLP Anchor... An anchor triggers a reaction in the mind body... we all know the symbol of water... and that water cleanses, detoxes, purifies and washes away... a pool of water can be refreshing and relaxing

Return to the image of the beach**...** I want you to return to the daydream of the warm sunny beach... you are walking down the beach... you can see the crystal clear, warm water... it looks so refreshing... inviting...

You relax... not a care in the world, stress free, carefree, deeply relaxed... just as if you were on a wonderful vacation...

you can imagine yourself going for a relaxing dip in the warm water... perhaps just floating and drifting... care-free, stress-free so completely relaxed.

Imagine that you can feel the warmth of the water soaking into your body... into your muscles, into every fiber, tissue, nerve and into every cell. Its swishing and swirling... clearing and cleansing... detoxing the body... detoxing the organs...organ systems... it soothes and calms any inflammation of the nerves...restores and refreshes the nervous systems...

clearing away any old cellular memory of pain or discomfort... washing, clearing every cell, cellular memory, fiber, nerve and muscle... flushing any blocks to your complete wellness... letting go... releasing it all... clearing cleansing... washing it all away.

Once again... imagine the magical drains on the very ends of your toes... the water flushes, clears and simply leaves the body thru these magical drains on the ends of your toes... until it gone. Completely cleared away...

I want you to now picture a bottle of drinking water... crystal clear, cool, refreshing... you like the taste of water and drink plenty of water... as you drink the water, it flushes and washes away painful inflammation... washes away the symptoms of crps... clearing... cleansing... washes away fatigue and tiredness... washing way brain fog... as you drink the water... you feel calm, relaxed, refreshed... completely renewed.

as it clears away the old, it brings in the new fresh energy... fresh new vitality... energy... life force energy flows freely through your mind and body... restoring... refreshing... new vitality...new energy... health and well-being... mentally, physically, emotionally and spiritually renewed.

You drink plenty of water... you keep your body well hydrated... when you drink the water you are free of CRPS pain or any symptoms... you feel calm and relaxed, free of anxiety, ... relaxed...
you are full of energy and vitality... you remember to drink the water.

Your subconscious mind now uses the symbol of water to clear and cleanse your mind and body... when you drink the water you are free of crps pain or discomfort... free of CRPS symptoms...

When you drink the water, you are...free of anxiety, you feel relaxed, calm, refreshed and restored of vital life force healing energy.
 Your subconscious has been given the symbol of water... it is your natural way to relax... stress-free calm and relaxed when you drink the water

---

Take a moment and practice Role Modeling again... only this time picture your life the way you would like it to be...

Pause for as long as you like to imagine your heart's desire... the future you want for yourself where you can see yourself successful...

financially prosperous... healthy... everything you always dreamed of... get a clear image... you may want to use someone as a role model to model this image after...

NOW... Imagine yourself stepping into this new you- a new life.

Picture yourself once again walking down the beach... use all your senses to place yourself in this favorite place you have created... this is your inner sanctuary... a place of healing... a mental escape where you can go to relax whenever you choose... by simply breathing... relaxing... and using your imagination to daydream... your subconscious mind knows this place... this healing sanctuary you have created.

You have finished this healing therapy, you might not understand exactly how all of this works... but just know that your subconscious mind... the most powerful part of your mind... knows what to do with the healing suggestions, the symbols and images that it has been given to heal your mind and body.

The more that you consistently listen to this recording, the more powerful the healing is. Your mind and body respond to the healing images, techniques and suggestions to return you to perfect health. Healed and Healthy today and from this day forward...

(READ THIS NEXT SECTION IN A LOUDER, STRONGER, COMMANDING VOICE)**

You Will Now Awaken And Return To Your Alert State Of Mind – Open Your Eyes

I want you to begin to awaken... be alert... Come back into your surroundings... and your body... On the count of 3- you will be wide awake and alert. 1.... 2 and 3 wide awake now.

(PAUSE AND READ)- if this is your bedtime… you will allow the recording to shut-off and return to peaceful sleep, awakening in the morning at your given time feeling well rested, energized ready to start your day… completely free of pain or discomfort.

STOP RECORDING - THE END OF SCRIPT

Module 11: The Power Of Remembered Wellness

Remembered Wellness

Dr Benson was a pioneer in mind-body medicine and founder of The Mind-Body Institute at the prestigious Massachusetts General Hospital. He authored several books; *The Relaxation Response, The Mind-body Effect,* and T*imeless Healing: the Power and Biology of Belief,* first published in 1995.

Remembered Wellness is a mental exercise, where the person taps into their memory to mentally return to a state of wellness before injury or illness ever occurred thus triggering the body's natural self-healing mechanism. The body is recovering its master blueprint of wellness in its memory of wholeness. When you use this technique, you are simply reminding the body of something it already knows, it remembers the state of wellness and has the ability to return to that state of wellness as Dr Benson's research has proven.

Some people think of the *Remembered Wellness* technique as being similar to the placebo effect where a person believes in the healing effects of a drug or therapy treatment and the healing comes to pass, even though the placebo pill is merely a sugar pill and has no medicinal value.

> ***"Whether it is pre-injury memory or the placebo-effect, an internal healing mechanism that cannot be medically explained is triggered in the person" - Dr Herbert Benson MD***

Dr Benson states in his book "all of us have the ability to remember the calm and confidence associated with health and happiness, but not just in an emotional or psychologically soothing way. This memory is also physical." Dr Benson concludes by writing "To me, the simple act of conjuring *remembered wellness* is more powerful than taking a pill called a placebo."

Dr Benson's Remembered Wellness technique is an exercise in Neural Retraining Therapy that was before its time. The technique literally flips a switch in the brain returning the mind and body to a state of prior wellness much like neuroscientist, Dr Norman Doidge MD pioneered in his neuroscience discoveries into brain neuroplasticity to "unlearn" behavioral patterns and healed his own illness.

The flow of life can be moving along and then something happens that disrupts that flow and that event gets frozen in time, stored in the memory. Instead of staying stuck in that moment, you can use techniques in Neural Retraining, techniques like *Remembered Wellness* to reframe the past differently to replace the memory of the event, injury or illness with a memory of wellness.

How To Use The Remembered Wellness Technique

Let's say I fall and injure my knee, instead of remembering the fall, pain (emotion) and injury, I want to replay the event in my mind (with no emotion) and envision myself walking along coming to the place where the injury occurred, and instead of remembering the fall (emotion, shock, stress), I imagine myself continuing to walk right through that time and space free from the fall, continuing on with what I was doing, as if the fall and injury never happened.

In a relaxed meditative state of mind, the level of time-space is suspended, I am returning to the time of the injury, and seeing it differently, I am reframing in my mind the entire event thus changing the outcome.

In your mind, you progress through the event as if it never happened, so you are not getting frozen or stuck in the injury mindset. As you mentally imagine this, you are returning your mind and body to a state of wellness. You are reframing in the mind and body how it was before the injury, before the illness, before the moment where the flow of health and wellness was disrupted.

Your mind and body know how to do this. You simply need to do the technique-repeatedly over 21-30 days to create a new neuropathway for positive change.

I have used this technique on myself and with therapy clients, not only for injury or illness but also for smoking cessation to return the smoker to a mental state before the smoking habit and nicotine addiction. Most people using Neural Retraining techniques to quit cigarettes, quit without withdrawal symptoms. Their mind and body remember what it is like to be a non-smoker – and non-smokers do not experience withdrawal symptoms. It's simply imagining a different outcome in a particular moment in time. Its Dr Benson's remembered wellness.

Remember the research of Dr Andrew Newberg discussed in the opening chapter of my book, which has shown that the body reacts to images in the imagination as if they are real. The subconscious mind has no mechanism to tell real from unreal. The Lemon Taste Test in the book gives a perfect example of this.

Let's face it these are amazing discoveries; and we are just beginning to tap into the power of our brain's influence on the mind and body in what Dr Benson calls "timeless healing." The potential to tap into the healing power that comes from connecting to that original state of wellness, what our mind holds as our master blueprint of wellness, is really only the beginning. There is more to discover and explore about what are mind-brain-body is capable of achieving.

PRACTICE EXERCISE: REMEMBERED WELLNESS

I gave the example of falling and injuring a knee, roleplay your event in the same way, as if the event never happened and you go on with your day. The subconscious mind will know what to do with the imagery. In psychology, this is called reframing, Dr Benson successfully used this technique "Remembered Wellness" for reprogramming your mental perception of an injury/trauma and bring your mind back to a state of wholeness, as if the injury/illness never occurred.

Start by getting into in to a relaxed meditative, quiet state of mind. Take 3-4 deep cleansing breaths, exhaling fully to relax the mind and body. Use the Inner Sanctuary imagery to allow the mind to daydream and escape for a few moments. We will be using the Role Modeling technique in this exercise. Use your role modeling images from previous exercises of a strong, vibrant healthy happy YOU.

Use your memory to go back in time to review the injury or illness event (without emotion, simply review it).

You will be reframing the event in your visualization so you are completely changing the event to make it have a positive outcome… as if the injury/event never happened. If you never experienced any pain or illness from the event. Make the imagery have a positive outcome.

INSTRUCTIONS: 2 different mini-meditations using remembered wellness.

1) **Morning Zen**: To reframe neuropathways, you will do this exercise daily each morning for the next 21-30 days to reframe in the brain the injury/illness. It should only be a brief 10 minute "reframing" visualization each day- preferable at the same time

of day where you envision yourself healthy and well, as if the injury/illness never occurred.

2) Evening Zen: To create new neuropathways to build self-confidence, where you know you have the ability to overcome life's obstacles, be successful, know joy and happiness- you will do this exercise in the afternoon/evening:

We use the Role Modeling Memory exercise: once again use your relaxation meditation skills to relax and envisions the strong vibrant image of yourself healthy and well.

Now use 2 memories in your visualization: 1) A time you succeeded at something, felt proud and self-confident you achieved a goal. You were very happy and pleased with yourself. 2) A time when you were wonderfully happy- joyous. Something/ event made you very happy, you were filled with jubilant enthusiasm and joy.

In the meditation, you actually bring that feeling of joy and happiness into your mind and body. With each breath you fill up with these emotions. Feel the self-confidence of achieving a goal or overcoming an obstacle. And make this role modeling image strong, powerful, successful, healthy (free of injury/illness) and full of vibrant joy and happiness!

Age does not matter in the memory exercise it can be something from decades ago. You will perform these mini "remembered wellness" role modeling mediations over the next 21-30-days.

Reading Suggestions: *Timeless Healing; the power and biology of belief* By Dr Herbert Benson MD (any of the books by Dr Benson)

Module 12: Therapy Script- Remembered Wellness

A Healing Script for Remembered Wellness
By Carol Charland   ~ All copyrights reserved 2023

Follow the instructions for recording the scripts.

PLEASE DO NOT LISTEN TO RECORDING WHILE DRIVING THE CAR

Get into a quiet place where you will not be disturbed, relax using your imagination to escape into a daydream of a beautiful garden in springtime. Let your mind and body do all the work for you.

(START RECORDING SCRIPT HERE)

Begin to use your imagination to tap into the power of your subconscious mind... relax by taking in three deep cleansing breaths, exhaling fully into a peaceful state of relaxation. Put all other thoughts aside for the time being and simply escape into the daydream. With each breath you relax more and more fully... all the stress and tension leave your mind and body.

Imagine the most beautiful, majestic garden before you with a pathway full of beautiful blooming flowers... you can see a bubbling water fountain up ahead with crystal clear bubbling water flowing... sparkling in the sunshine like diamonds... the sky is clear soft blue color with white fluffy clouds... a warm breeze is blowing through your hair... and you walk along the garden pathway.

You can feel the warmth of the sunshine on your face... radiant golden beams of sunshine surround you in pure golden light... relaxing, feeling stress-free as you walk along this garden path.

With each exhale of your breath imagine you can send the golden beams of solar radiance like a warm soothing wave... down from the top of your head... to the tips of your toes... surrounding you with golden radiance... a relaxing, soothing, comforting wave of energy infuses your mind, body and spirit... and you relax.

The solar radiance clears the aura surrounding your physical body... it clears blockages from the meridian pathways... it heals, clears, aligns and activates your chakra energy system... bringing beautiful radiant life force energy or "Chi" to your entire being...

Imagine... It's a beautiful spring day... you breathe in the fresh air of springtime and send it through your mind and body... You know that springtime is a time of new beginnings...and a fresh start.

It's a fresh start for you in your life... send this message through your mind and body... simply breathing in the fresh spring air and relaxing into the comfort of your own body... a fresh new start... new beginnings...

Ahead on the garden path you see a swing in a big strong oak tree... imagine sitting down in the swing to rest a while... you remember what it is like to swing on a swing set... such a stress-free, care-free feeling, it brings a smile to your face... it's fun to swing...

Imagine gently swinging back and forth on the swing... feeling the warmth of the sunshine.... Breathing in the fresh air of springtime. stress-free, care-free and relaxed.

You feel the warm sunshine on your face... relaxing all the muscles across your forehead... around your eyes... and like a warm wave of relaxation... it flows down your face into jaw and throat...

Let the wave of warm sunshine flow down your neck and into your arms... your hands and fingers... right out thru your fingertips... letting go of any old stale energy... relaxing now

Imagine filling your spine with beautiful sparkling golden beams of sunlight... from the base of your spine... all the way up to the base of your skull... a golden ray of sunlight fills your spine... imagine it aligns and heals your spine, heals nerves and your nervous system...

And now... the warm wave of golden beams of sunlight moves down into your chest and abdomen... relaxing muscles...

As you breathe it moves down into your hips... down your legs into feet and toes... right out through the ends of your toes... letting go of stress and tension.... Letting it all go now.

Breathe and relax...let your mind and body escape into the daydream... a beautiful spring day... a fresh start and new beginnings...

While you relax... I want you to go back into your memory... back to a time BEFORE your injury or illness... (or back to a time BEFORE the stressful event) when you were completely well.

I want you to remember what the feeling of complete wellness feels like... remember everything about it... there was an absence of any illness or symptoms... you were free of illness or symptoms... both mentally and physically well.

Take a moment and picture yourself BEFORE... where you are completely well. See yourself in your mind... BEFORE...

and completely well. As if you have always been well.

Repeat it silently to yourself: as if I have always been well.

Now make this image of yourself very strong, bold, beautiful, healthy... breathe strength into this image...

ADD aliveness and color to the image...

ADD emotion to this image... remember how wonderful it feels to be healthy and well.

ADD the feeling of "WHOLENESS" ... whole-person wellness... that every broken part of you is healed, as if you were never broken. That's right. as if you were never broken.

Repeat it silently to yourself "***As if I were never broken***".
Feel the sensation of aliveness...and you are whole once again.

ADD love, joy and happiness to this new self—image.
Make it feel alive... beautiful... strong... and you are strong once again. You know it... you feel it deep inside... the message is being written on every cell, fiber, muscle and nerve... its being written in your mind and body... I am strong... I am whole.

Return to the daydream of the spring day... the garden... you are swinging back and forth on the swing... relaxed... stress-free, care-free... swinging back and forth...feeling the warmth of sunshine... breathing in the fresh spring air...

Now picture the strong beautiful image of yourself once again... see it in your mind before you.

I want you to use your imagination... imagine you are melting and merging into this new self-image... when you were completely well... before any injury or illness... before any stressful event...

Simply step into this image you created of yourself "whole" ... strong... whole once again... as if you have always been strong and whole... as if you have always been completely well.

Melt and merge in the warm sunlight... from the top of your head... to the tips of your toes... into this new self-image....

Return to wellness... imagine your mind and body flipping the switch... back to a state of remembered wellness... where you are completely well.

Take a moment... pause... feel it in your body... (pause)
Feel it in your mind... (pause) feel it deep within to the core of your very soul... this is who you are... completely well... its who you were always meant to be.

And you can relax now your work is done... imagine yourself walking along the garden pathway... no blocks... no obstacles in your way... see ahead a bright future... complete wellness... in all ways...

Every day you feel better and better... in every way.

Bask in the feeling... healed and healthy.

Your subconscious mind knows what to do with the images, symbols and suggestions it has been given to return you to a state of complete wellness... it remembers... it knows how to do this... and it does it... now.

Every day you will notice subtle but amazing changes taking place ... feeling completely well once again as if you have always been well.

You have activated your own inner self-healing mechanism...

As you walk along the garden path, you'll notice a sign that reads: ***Garden Of Strength.***

You will begin to plant seeds of strength in your subconscious mind... that enable you to achieve your heart's desire. to heal the mind and body... and achieve your highest level of health and wellbeing...

Imagine you are planting flowers in the spring garden of strength...

First you will plant a beautiful **red flower...** this brings to your life balance and harmony... it brings stability in your life... it grounds your energy giving you strength and the personal power to cope and manage with any stress that comes your way. Like the roots of a tree that strengthens the tree... this is the root of your life ... it will grow and expand in miraculous ways.

Next plant an **orange flower**... this plants self-love, caring for yourself, and it's the motivation and the desire to achieve your goals in life.... It activates your creativity and stabilizes your emotional and mental body... it brings love, joy and happiness in your life.

Now plant a **yellow flower...** this is the seat of the soul... it connects you to all that is... it builds your self-confidence in your own ability to achieve wellness, success in life and most importantly to achieve your life purpose... it activates all your natural God-given skills and abilities to succeed in your life purpose...

Next you plant an **emerald, green plant**... this expands your capacity to love and be loved... and gives you the power of healing transformations- emotionally, mentally, physically and spiritually. It activates the healer within… your natural self-healing mechanism. It is the purest form of unconditional love being sent to you now.

A beautiful silvery **blue colored flower** is next… this opens up the channels of communication and self-expression for you… it is self-expression… to be who you are meant to be in this life…

You plant a deep **Indigo blue colored flower**… that brings you the power of intuition and universal knowledge… it activates your sense of imagination, creativity and foresight… You intuitively know and make right decisions to heal and live your best life… It brings guidance in all things to you.

Next in your garden of strengths… you plant a **majestic purple flower**… this connects you to all things in the universe… God, your higher power…it connects you to your true soul purpose. It mends all the broken pieces of your mind… your body… your soul… and brings you back to a state of "wholeness." It brings healing to your life in its entirety.

Finally, you plant a **beautiful white flower**… that wraps you in a safe cocoon of soothing calm… it is your shield of protection… it is always there for you… protecting you… guiding you… to your best life.

Take a moment and look out over your garden… you planted seeds of deep inner strengths…along with your natural God-given skills and abilities… you now possess everything you need to heal and achieve your goals in life… and you do.

Imagine walking down the garden path before you… see it is a clear path… there are no blocks or obstacles in your way… you successfully achieve your goals… you are on a clear path to a bright future.

Walking along the pathway... stress-free, care-free... healed and healthy not a care in the world... feeling in complete balance and harmony with all that is...

You are better able to control stress now...you relax naturally... and have heathy coping mechanisms. You let stress bounce off from you like a red-rubber ball...

You can handle anything that comes your way... in a calm relaxed manner...

You take good care of your health... you are the picture of wellness.

I want you to imagine on the garden pathway you can see a magnificent water fountain... bubbling... crystal clear water .... sparkling like diamonds in the sunlight...

I want you to imagine in your hand... you have a coin... I want you to put a label on the coin of a goal you want to achieve... or a heart's desire... whatever you want to bring into your life.

Picture the coin in your hand with the label on it... you have heard this water fountain is a called the fountain of miracles... when you toss a coin in the fountain... it brings to you what you desire...

See yourself tossing the coin with the label on it... into the fountain... and as splash of beautiful rainbow colors surround you... bringing to you your heart's desire... you feel joy and happiness... and a sense of satisfaction and contentment in life now...

Imagine what it feels like to have that in your life... picture it for a moment... acknowledge that the coin will appear in your life when the time is right...

Once again you picture yourself on the magical garden pathway basking in the warmth of the solar radiance… beams of golden sunlight… breathing in the fresh air of springtime and new beginnings…

You have accomplished such an amazing number of wonderful things today… This is a new beginning for you… like the spring day… it's a fresh start…

Picture yourself… just as you truly want it to be… and so it is.

You might not understand exactly how all of this works… but just know your subconscious mind knows what to do with the pictures and symbols given to it… to help you achieve your goals.

On the count of 3- you will be WIDE AWAKE AND ALERT---

    1- Open your eyes and see the room around you
    2- Move about… feel back in your body
    3- You are wide awake and alert now…

(PAUSE AND READ) If this is time you are sleeping, you will turn off the recording and return to sound peaceful sleep throughout the night. Awaken in the morning feeling refreshed, energized and ready to start your day…

END OF SCRIPT.   STOP RECORDING.

Module 13: The 30-Day Plan

The Pain Survival Tool Kit

The book is divided into learning modules and offers a step-by-step teaching guide to practice the NLP Neurolinguistic retraining techniques for pain relief. You can create your own customized *Pain Survival Tool Kit* by utilizing this plan.

Below you will find the priority steps to getting started on this program:

- **Priority 1: (Script #1)** Read through the Recordable Meditation Therapy Script(s) and set up your recording device to record it so you can begin listening to Script #1 immediately. Record and listen to the Recordable Meditation Therapy Script for CRPS (script #1) recording for 30 days. At bedtime, simply fall to sleep listening to it and let it fill your mind, body and soul with the healing messages for pain relief. After the 30-day period, listen to the audio recording a few times a week then perhaps once a month for maintaining the changes you have achieved.
- **Script #2:** You can listen to the Remembered Wellness script as often as you would like to begin the program, I recommend in the mornings to restore and reinforces wellness.
- **The Havening Technique:** Repeatedly use the Havening technique over the next 30 days to release the root cause of the injury and trauma causing pain. Use it for any new stress you may experience as well as physical and emotional symptoms.
- **Pain Relief Techniques**: Choose a few of your favorite NLP pain anesthesia techniques for pain relief and use the same technique daily to manage pain levels. These techniques retrain

the mind-brain-body, paving new neuropathways, switching from pain mode to pain-free. You can record these mini-exercises to listen to for quick pain relief. Remember, the more you use these on a daily basis, the more immediate the pain relief and the more beneficial they become in retraining your brain to be pain-free.

- **Role Modeling & The Swish Technique:** Start using the Role Modeling and Swish Technique to release specific trauma, pain and symptoms. You can use it for stress and anxiety or any behavior pattern you wish to change. You may want to record the step-by-step guide to the techniques, so you automatically follow each step of the technique. Repetition of these exercises is key to successfully paving new neural pathways.
- **Limbic Brain Reset: Practice Stress Control**: Use *The Inner Sanctuary* and *Progressive Relaxation* techniques for natural relaxation and stress control on a daily basis to help calm the nervous system and shuts off the pain alarm.
- **Selfcare Strategies:** Set up a Pacing Activity Program. Find a pacing pain app you like that you will use to set up for pacing activities. You can avoid over-activity pain flareups by using the Pacing technique.
- **Diet:** Research the pain-friendly diet suggestions to incorporate into your lifestyle. Consult your physician or a nutritionist for an anti-inflammatory, clean eating diet plan.
- **Create your Self-care plan for the week.** Schedule regular time periods for self-care activities. Get creative by including hobbies, walks out in nature and CAM Complimentary-Alternative therapies to nourish and soothe the soul.
- **Support Group**: Living with chronic pain and illness is not easy. We all need help and support. Find a local or online group that supports your needs.

Resources

You will find listed below some of my favorite resources that helped me in my quest for understanding and managing chronic pain and illness.

Books

Dr Candace Pert, MD "Molecules of Emotion" and "Your Body Is Your Subconscious Mind".

Dr Larry Dossey, MD "Healing Words; The Power of Prayer & The Practice of Medicine"

Dr Larry Dossey, MD "Healing Beyond The Body: Medicine & The Infinite Reach of The Mind"

Dr Norman Doidge MD "The Brains Way Of Healing"

Dr Andrew Newberg MD and Mark Robert Waldman "Words Can Change Your Brain"

Dr Herbert Benson MD "The Relaxation Response" and "Timeless Healing".

Dr Jacob Teitelbaum MD book: "The Fatigue and Fibromyalgia Solution" and "From Fatigued Too Fantastic"

Dr Lawrence Afrin MD Book: "Never Bet Against Occam" Mast Cell Activation Disorder

Toni Bernhard "How To Be Sick" and "How To Live Well" (ACT Therapy) Toni Bernhard authors articles for Psychology Today about living life to the fullest with chronic pain and illness. You can find her inspirational posts online at Psychology Today.

Organizations

RSDSA Organization   www.rsds.org   The leading organization for CRPS~RSD.

RSD CANADA Organization www.rsdcanada.org
For Grace: www.forgrace.org An organization promoting care for women facing persistent pain

Burning Nights UK Organization: www.burningnightscrps.org

Dysautonomia International Organization: Information on Dysautonomia and POTS Postural Orthostatic Tachycardia Syndrome www.dysautonomiainternational.org

LDN Research Trust Organization: LDN or Low Dose Naltrexone: An opiate-free lifechanging medication used for chronic pain, reducing inflammation and boosting the immune system. For more information on the conditions that have been remarkably helped by LDN find clinical studies on their webpage. www.ldnresearchtrust.org

Institute For Chronic Pain Organization: Find information on Central Sensitization Syndrome as a com-morbid condition to pain syndromes. Hypervigilance anxiety pain-induced. Brain inflammation and sensory overload issues. www.instituteforchronicpain.org

Medical

Dr Pradeep Chopra MD: Leading Pain Management expert in Pawtucket RI. A Pain Specialist, Graduate of Harvard Medical, Professor at Brown Medical School, Brown University. Many of his RSDSA Organization Conference videos are on YouTube so you can watch the entire conference on CRPS, pain management and treatment of co-morbid conditions.

Dr Philip Getson DO: Dr Getson offers whole person treatment with holistic- complimentary therapy options as well as traditional medical care. You can watch his Conference videos on YouTube for the management and treatment of pain syndromes.

Dr Robert Hooshmand MD: Research articles The 4F's Diet www.rsdrx.com

Dr Robert J Schwartzman MD, Drexel University: Article "Systemic Complications of CRPS"

Dr Lawrence Afrin MD   www.armonkmed.com   MCAD/ Mast Cell Activation Disorder

Carol Charland-Cliche

Carol Charland-Cliche holds a Diploma in CAM Complimentary ~ Alternative Medicine, an NLP Neurolinguistics Pain Management Practitioner and a Certified Clinical Hypnotherapist since 1998. She is a member of IACT, The International Association of Counselors and Therapists.

As a Pain Management Practitioner, Carol has a unique understanding of persistent pain, better than most author-therapists. She has CRPS- Complex Regional Pain Syndrome rated the highest known pain syndrome on the McGill Pain Scale. She knows the struggles of living a life in persistent pain. She has written the therapeutic pain relief programs not only from her expertise as a CAM Pain Management Practitioner that has successfully helped hundreds of clients over the years but also from her own life experience of living in persistent pain.

Carol triumphed over CRPS and is currently in remission. She went on to develop the revolutionary new 4R's Neuroplastic Healing System based on the latest neuroscience discoveries in neuroplasticity and using her own life experience searching for effective opiate-free pain relief for CRPS. She offers a variety of *Retrain Your Brain* wellness books, online courses and private wellness coaching via Zoom online.

Carol lives in beautiful Southern Coastal Maine. She enjoys time with her grandchildren and the beautiful Maine beaches, mountains and lakes where the motto is "life the way it should be." When Carol is not writing books, she loves to walk the beach with her little diva canine, Daisy collecting sea glass that has washed up on the shores from around the world.

www.carolcharland.com

Book Acknowledgements

To my family, friends and therapy clients:
Thank you for your continued support and encouragement in publishing my life's work.

Patricia Wilson: Proofreading & Editing Services

Indie Graphics: Book Cover / paperback

Katherine Mayfield: A special acknowledgement for Katherine Mayfield, Author of the award-winning memoir *"The box of daughter; A guide to recovery from bullying"* and *"Stand your ground: how to cope with a dysfunctional family"* I am grateful for her expertise and motivation in helping me become an Independent Author and Publisher.

Made in the USA
Monee, IL
18 June 2023

36111525R00092